YOGA
YOUR HOME PRACTICE COMPANION

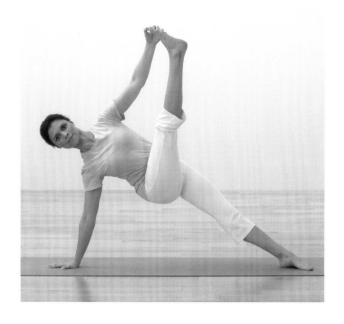

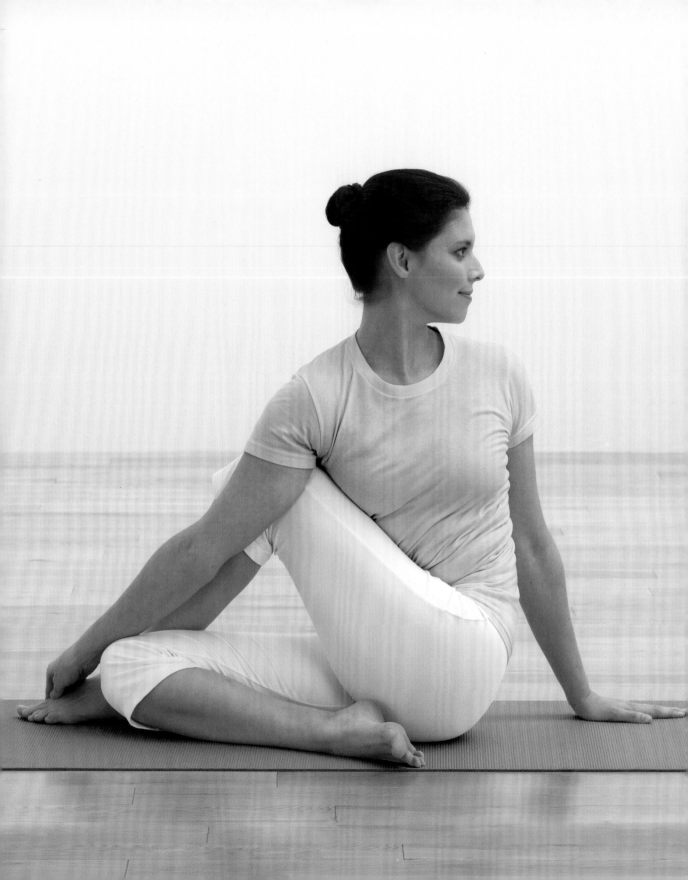

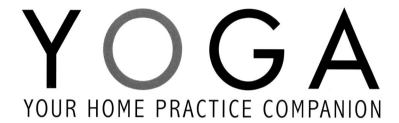

YOGA

YOUR HOME PRACTICE COMPANION

Sivananda Yoga Vedanta Center

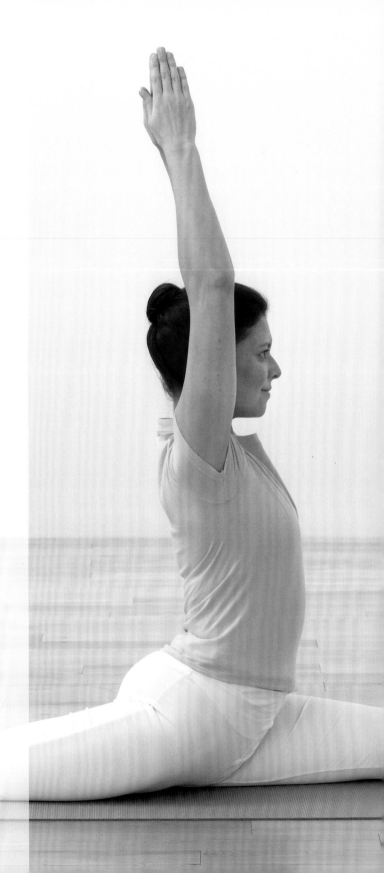

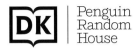

For H.H. Sri Swami Vishnudevananda

Authors for the Sivananda Yoga Vedanta Center

Swami Durgananda
Swami Sivasananda
Swami Kailasananda

SECOND EDITION
Senior Editors Cecile Landau & Kate Meeker
US Editor Megan Douglass
Senior Art Editor Glenda Fisher
Senior Jacket Designer Nicola Powling
Pre-producer, Production Rebecca Fallowfield
Producer Igrain Roberts
Managing Editor Stephanie Farrow
Managing Art Editor Christine Keilty

This American Edition, 2018
First American Edition, 2009
Published in the United States by DK Publishing
1450 Broadway, Suite 801, New York, NY 10018

Health warning
All participants in fitness activities must assume the
responsibility for their own actions and safety. If you have any
health problems or medical conditions, consult with your
physician before undertaking any of the activities set out in this
book. The information contained in this book cannot replace
sound judgement and good decision making, which can help
reduce risk of injury.

A catalog record for this book
is available from the Library of Congress.
ISBN: 978-1-4654-7318-9

Printed and bound in China

Sivananda Yoga Vedanta Center
www.sivananda.org

For the curious
www.dk.com

MIX
Paper from
responsible sources
FSC™ C018179

This book was made with Forest Stewardship
Council™ certified paper – one small step in
DK's commitment to a sustainable future.
For more information go to
www.dk.com/our-green-pledge

Contents

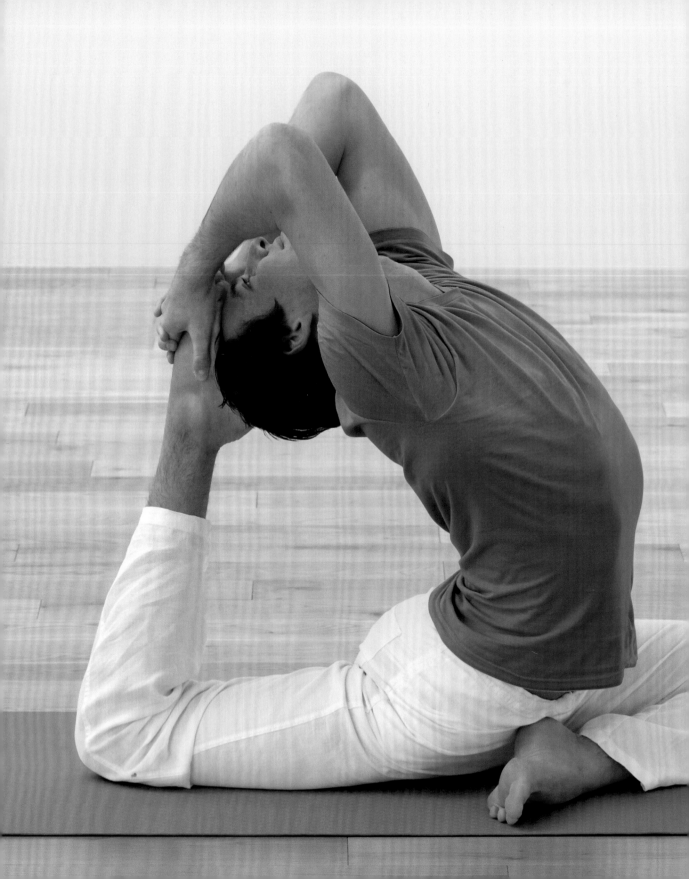

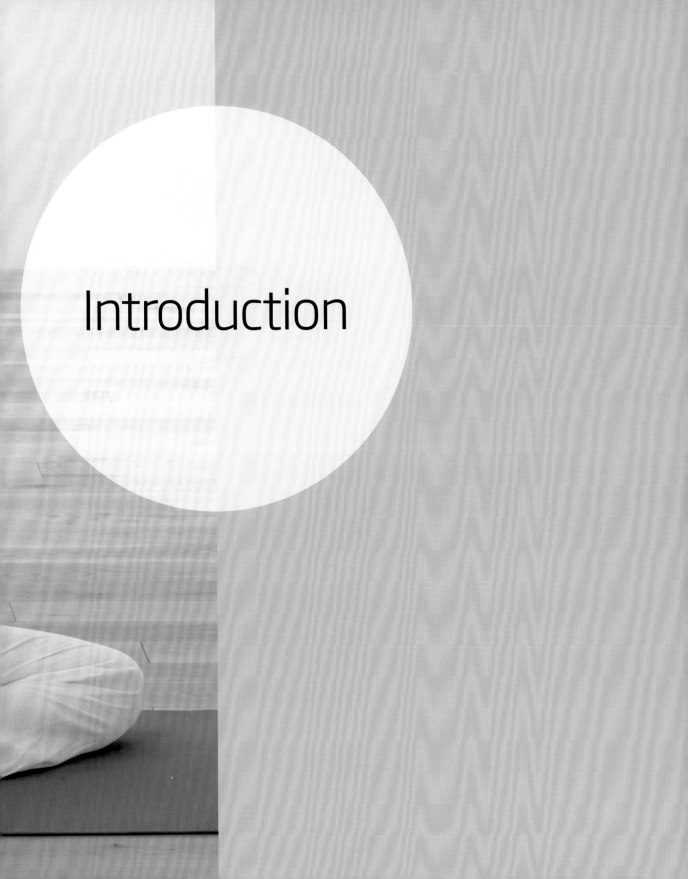

Introduction

An ancient guide to healthy living

Yoga is a centuries-old guide to healthy living developed by ancient Indian sages. With its unique blend of physical exercises, psychological insight, and philosophy, it can help you to bring your body, mind, and spirit into better balance. Yoga takes a holistic approach to life, enabling you to experience complete equilibrium inside and out.

Yoga for everyone

For centuries, yoga was open only to people who were ready to search for a teacher in India, and traditionally it only appealed to those willing to forego the life of a "householder," renouncing the world and living in seclusion. H.H. Swami Sivananda (1887–1963) and Swami Vishnudevananda (1927–1993) were among the first of the Indian yoga masters to make yoga accessible to anyone, no matter their background, age, or status, or where in the world they lived. In doing so, they helped to bring yoga to the West.

Swami Sivananda

Sri Swami Sivananda was a practicing doctor who was eager to do all he could to relieve human misery. In a search to ease his patients' physical and mental discomfort, he decided to look within himself. He began his quest by becoming a swami—a wandering monk—and after long years of secluded practice in the Himalayas, he attained mastery in yoga and meditation. Swami Sivananda went on to found the Divine Life Society in Rishikesh, in the Himalayas. Here, he trained students from many countries and various religions in a synthesis of the key paths of yoga, encompassing Hatha and Raja Yoga, Karma Yoga, Bhakti Yoga, and Jnana Yoga (see pp10–11). He also wrote more than 200 books in English explaining the most complex aspects of yoga in simple, practical terms.

Swami Vishnudevananda and the West

Swami Vishnudevananda was a close disciple of Swami Sivananda and adept in the practice of Hatha and Raja Yoga (see p10). In 1957, Swami Sivananda commanded him to "Go to the West, people are waiting."

"Yoga is a science perfected by the ancient seers of India, not of India merely, but of humanity as a whole. It is an exact science. It is a perfect, practical system of self-culture."

Swami Sivananda

With no means of support other than his faith and a remarkable energy, Swami Vishnudevananda traveled to North America, Europe, and many other parts of the world, where he became a pioneer in yoga, spreading the teachings of his master.

Swami Vishnudevananda founded the International Sivananda Yoga Vedanta Centers at the heart of many of the world's capital cities. Here, people are able to learn yoga as they go about their daily lives. Swami Vishnudevananda also established several ashrams (yoga retreats) in beautiful natural settings around the globe, from the forested mountains of Canada to Paradise Island in the Bahamas. He promoted yoga vacation programs, which offer people an opportunity to learn the yogic disciplines while enjoying a healthy and relaxing vacation.

After experiencing a vision during meditation, Swami Vishnudevananda felt compelled to start up a campaign for world peace, which became known as T.W.O., True World Order. It adopted the mottos, "United we live—divided we perish" and "Cross man-made borders with flowers and love, not with bombs and guns." Swami Vishnudevananda learned how to pilot a small plane and flew over many of the world's conflict zones, showering them with flowers and leaflets promoting the universal love taught by all the world's great religions. Two memorable flights took him over the Suez canal during the Sinai War in 1971 and over the Berlin Wall from West Germany to East Germany in 1983.

Teacher training

As part of his vision of yoga for world peace, Swami Vishnudevananda taught the first yoga teachers' training course in the West, in 1969. As well as offering a broad study of yoga philosophy, psychology, and teaching techniques, the four-week residential program focused on an intense personal practice of yoga and meditation. It is even more popular today than during Swami Vishnudevananda's lifetime. Since the training course was founded, more than 25,000 graduates from all walks of life and every continent have taken the yoga teachings of Swami Vishnudevananda and Swami Sivananda back into their own communities.

The defining feature of this approach to yoga is its simplicity: regardless of age, physique, and walk of life, anyone can benefit from this step-by-step guide to asana (exercise), pranayama (breathing), relaxation, diet, positive thinking, and meditation. These key teachings are outlined in the chapters of this book to help you, too, to experience this ancient way of bringing balance into every aspect of your life.

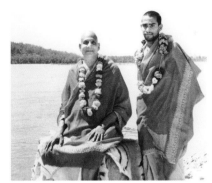

A JOURNEY BEGINS
Shortly before his departure to the West, Swami Vishnudevananda stands beside his master, Swami Sivananda.

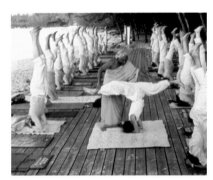

TRAINING THE TEACHERS
An asana class during a teachers' training course in Nassau, The Bahamas. Swami Vishnudevananda works with a student.

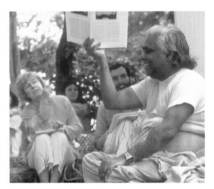

PIONEERING WORK
Swami Vishnudevananda was one of the first Indian master yogis to spread the teaching of yoga across the western world.

What is yoga?

Traditionally, there are four paths of yoga. Although each of them is a complete discipline in itself, it is best not to follow one path only. Combining the four practices helps the emotional, intellectual, and physical aspects of your life to develop in harmony.

The four paths of yoga

Of the four yogic paths, in the West only one is generally well-known and widely practiced—the physical and mind-focusing path of Hatha and Raja Yoga, which includes postures and breathing exercises.

HATHA AND RAJA YOGA This is the yogic path of body and mind control. It is best known for its practical aspects, particularly its asanas (postures) and pranayama (breathing exercises). This path teaches ways of controlling the body and mind, including silent meditation, and its practices gradually transform the energy of the body and mind into spiritual energy. This path suits people who are looking for inner and outer transformation.

KARMA YOGA This is the yogic path of action and you practice it when you act selflessly, without thinking about success or reward. This path is valued for purifying the heart and reducing the influence of the ego on your words, actions, and interaction with others. Practicing Karma Yoga is the best way to prepare yourself for silent meditation (see pp202–204). It suits people with an active, outgoing temperament.

BHAKTI YOGA This is the yogic path of devotion. It involves prayer, worship, and ritual, including chanting and singing devotional songs, and those who practice it eventually come to experience God as the embodiment of love. This yogic path has great appeal for people who are emotional by nature.

JNANA YOGA This is the yogic path of wisdom or knowledge, and it involves studying the philosophy of Vedanta—one of the six classical Indian philosophies. It teaches ways to examine the self and analyze human nature. The goal of this form of yoga is to recognize the Supreme Self in yourself and in all beings. This path is best suited to intellectual people, and is considered by many to be the most challenging path.

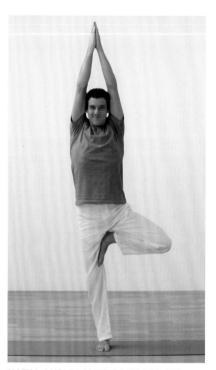

HATHA AND RAJA YOGA IN ACTION
This path includes the practice of asanas. Each asana requires a specific balance of posture, breathing, and relaxation.

The eight steps of Hatha and Raja Yoga

This path was codified by the ancient sage Patanjali in his *Yoga Sutras* as an eight-step training system for body and mind, which he called Ashtanga Yoga (in Sanskrit, *ashta* is "eight" and *anga* "division" or "limb"). The steps purify body and mind until enlightenment occurs.

1 YAMA Sets out the actions from which yogis should refrain. It advocates living a life of non-violence and truthfulness, sublimating sexual energy, not stealing, and not accepting gifts or bribes.

2 NIYAMA Details the actions a yogi should do. It advocates external and internal cleanliness, contentment, self-discipline, study of spiritual literature, and devotion to God. Together, the yamas and niyamas form a highly moral code of ethical conduct. Following them makes the mind more positive and purifies it, ready for deep meditation.

3 ASANA The third step relates to posture. The 12 basic asanas and their variations prepare the body for the meditative poses that are used in steps 6, 7, and 8.

4 PRANAYAMA The fourth step concerns control of prana or life energy. This is achieved by doing deep-breathing exercises, which include practicing breath retention (see pp182–185).

5 PRATYAHARA Steps 3 and 4 project the practitioner into a world of intense inner perception. Step 5 teaches how to stabilize this withdrawal of the senses as a preparation for concentration.

6 DHARANA In this step, concentration, the mind is fixed on an imaginary or real object to the exclusion of other thoughts. This is the key practice in all yoga meditation techniques (see pp200–204).

7 DHYANA Step 6 leads to step 7, meditation. This uninterrupted flow of thought waves has been compared to oil flowing in an unbroken stream from one container to another.

8 SAMADHI The final step happens effortlessly as, during meditation, the mind is absorbed into Absolute Consciousness, beyond all the usual states of waking, dreaming, and deep sleep (see p198).

"You can have calmness of mind at all times by the practice of yoga. You can have restful sleep. You can have increased energy, vigor, vitality, longevity, and a high standard of health. You can turn out efficient work within a short space of time. You can have success in every walk of life."

Swami Sivananda

The yogic path to well-being

Swami Vishnudevananda taught five easy principles of yoga, all of which are explained in different chapters in this book. They bring together the often-complex philosophies and teachings of India's ancient yogis in a form that is easy to understand and simple to adapt to everyday life, wherever you live in the world.

The five principles of yoga

If you follow these five easy principles, said Swami Vishnudevananda, you will improve your physical and mental health and deepen your connection with the spiritual aspects of life.

Proper exercise

Asanas (see pp42–169) rejuvenate the whole body. They work primarily on the spine and central nervous system. The spine gains in strength and flexibility, and circulation is stimulated, bringing nutrients and oxygen to all the cells of the body. Asanas increase motion in the joints and flexibility in muscles, tendons, and ligaments. They massage internal organs, boosting their function.

Proper breathing

Pranayama (see pp176–185) stimulates the energy reserves of the solar plexus, revitalizing body and mind. Regulating the breath helps to store prana, laying down reserves of strength and vitality. Deep, conscious breathing helps conquer depression and stress, and controlling prana—by controlling the breath—can relieve the symptoms of illness in a manner similar to acupuncture.

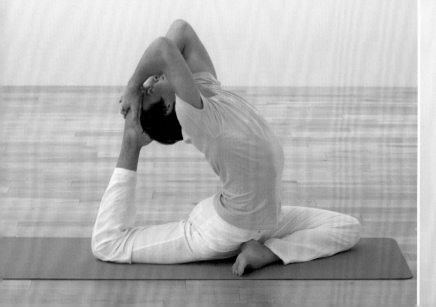

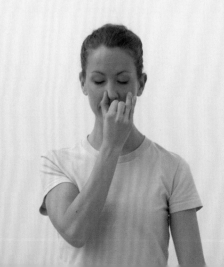

Proper relaxation

Deep relaxation (see pp186–195) works on three levels—physical, mental, and spiritual—and is the most natural way to re-energize body and mind. Regular relaxation acts like a car's cooling system, keeping the engine from over-heating and ensuring the vehicle functions efficiently. During the deep relaxation at the end of a yoga session, the body uses only enough prana to maintain vital metabolic activities. The rest of the energy gained during practice is stored.

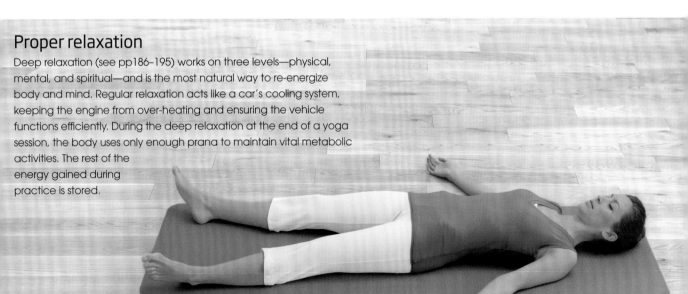

Proper diet

The yogic attitude to food (see pp208–249) is eat to live, not live to eat. Yogis choose foods with a positive effect on body and mind, and least negative effects on the environment and other creatures. A lacto-vegetarian diet is recommended—grains, pulses, fruits and vegetables, nuts, seeds, and dairy products—including plenty of plants. Fresh and unrefined foods are thought best, prepared simply, to preserve maximum nutrients.

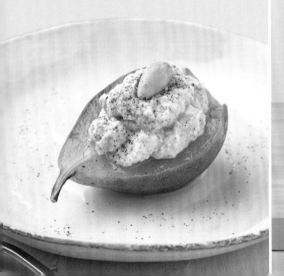

Positive thinking and meditation

Positive thinking and meditation (see pp198–207) are the yogic keys to peace of mind. Meditation techniques calm the mind and enhance focus. Regular meditation promotes physical and spiritual, as well as mental, well-being. Before meditation, yoga practitioners clear the mind of negative thoughts and feelings using concentration and positive-thinking exercises.

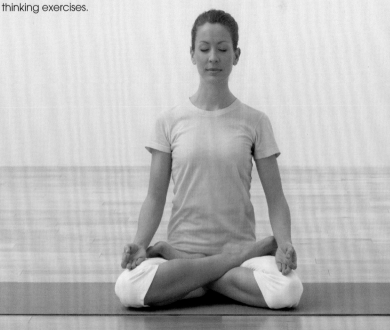

The Hatha Yoga Pradipika

The oldest surviving text on Hatha Yoga, the *Hatha Yoga Pradipika* is said to have been written down by Yogi Swatmarama in the 15th century, although it is derived from earlier sources. Despite being more than five centuries old, the advice given in this manual on postures, breathing exercises, and the philosophy of yoga is still relevant today, whether you are a beginner or a more experienced practitioner.

Selected extracts

These six extracts from the *Hatha Yoga Pradipika*—which translates as "Light on Hatha Yoga"—have been selected to inspire your practice. Commentaries suggest how to apply them to deepen your yoga experience.

Swatmarama Yogi, having saluted his own teacher, gives out the Hatha Vidya (knowledge) solely for the attainment of Raja Yoga. [12]

This passage stresses the importance of thinking of your practice as a way of controlling the mind—this is the path of Hatha and Raja Yoga (see p10). Many in the West regard asanas (see pp42–175) as a form of physical exercise only, but practicing them in this way is not to be recommended. It is impossible to master the mind without first controlling its physical counterpart, the body. This is what we seek to do when practicing postures. The connection between body and mind is one of the most fascinating aspects of yoga.

Asanas make one firm, free from disease, and light of limb. [17]

This explains how beneficial asana practice is. The "firmness" is seen in many ways, including improved alignment; increased resistance to heat, cold, hunger and thirst; and greater capacity for self-healing. Lightness of limb does not mean only physical weight (although asana practice does help to maintain an ideal weight), but the ability of asanas to raise the vibratory level of the body's energy. This is seen in movement: if someone with a large frame practices asanas, a new lightness appears in their movements.

Moderate diet is defined to mean taking pleasant and sweet food, leaving one-fourth of the stomach free, and offering the act up to Siva. I 58

Here, we are told that a moderate, nutritious, and light diet is key to success in yoga. Easily digested, fresh, vegetarian foods, simply cooked, are thought to be a good source of prana, or life force. Swami Sivananda advised that the way to be always happy is always to feel a little hungry.

When the breath wanders, i.e., is irregular, the mind is also unsteady, but when the breath is still, so is the mind, and the yogi lives long. So one should restrain the breath. II 2

Breath control is central to yoga: the term *Hatha* means "union of the sun (*Ha*) and the moon (*Tha*)," where sun and moon refer to inhalation and exhalation respectively. Both asanas and pranayama (see pp178–179) provide excellent training for the breath, which increases vital energy, fine-tunes the nervous system, and eventually leads to control of the mind.

He should gradually inhale the breath and as gradually exhale it. He should also restrain it gradually. II 18

This highlights the real hallmark of an accomplished practitioner of yoga. Strength and flexibility in postures are not by themselves a sign of progress. A smooth, rhythmical, balanced breath is. But never make any violent effort to control the breath in your yoga practice; this strains the nervous system.

The yogi succeeds by cheerfulness, perseverance, courage, true knowledge, firm belief in the words of the guru, and by abandoning bad company. I 16

Making yoga practice your own by having the right "knowledge" and "firm belief" (in the five principles, see pp12–13) opens the door to new friendships with like-minded people. The purpose of yoga is to shift your life force from a dormant or static state to a dynamic state. This requires perseverance, self-discipline, and courage.

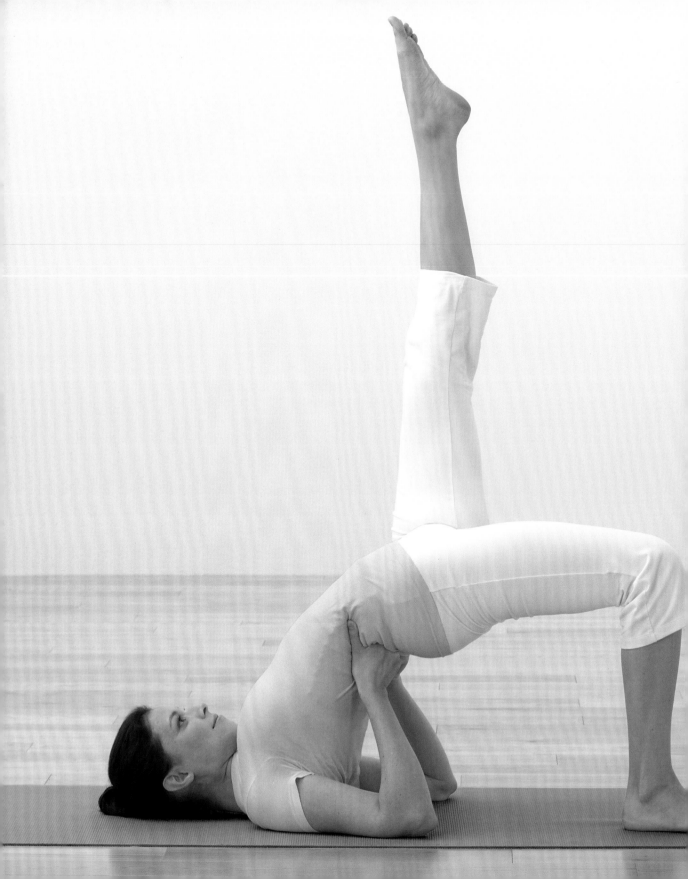

The Benefits of Yoga

Boosting self-healing

The human body is superbly intelligent. It manages to maintain an intricate physiological balance day and night, through every stage of life. Practicing yoga helps the body to maintain this complex balance, which boosts your capacity for self-healing.

The study of physiology shows that the nervous and the endocrine systems (see pp34–37) ensure that the body's other major systems, such as the digestive and respiratory systems, all cooperate in an "intelligent" way. The result is "homeostasis," derived from Greek and meaning "remaining the same." When homeostasis is achieved, there is perfect balance between the various body functions and, as long as the body has a regular supply of food and water and is not over-taxed physically, it tends naturally toward self-healing. Ancient yogis described a different but equally complex system of homeostasis in the body, based on a finely tuned balance of the five elements: earth, water, fire, air, and "ether," or space (see right). When these elements are in equilibrium, again body and mind tend toward self-healing.

The causes of disease

Why, then, does the body succumb to illness, even in parts of the world where there is no scarcity of food or water and where people do not have to do hard physical labor? According to yoga, the chief cause of disease lies in difficult emotions, such as anxiety, desire, anger, hatred, and jealousy. These disturb the body's natural balance and can lead to unhealthy lifestyle choices, from overeating to smoking. These, in turn, are factors in many diseases common in modern societies, from heart disease to diabetes.

Balancing the emotions

Practicing positive thinking and meditation (see pp196–207) makes it less likely that you will be affected by negative emotions and the lifestyle choices they lead to. But it is easier to meditate and think positively if you first pay attention to the body, practicing yoga asanas, or postures (see pp42–169), pranayama breathing exercises (see pp176–185), and relaxation (see pp186–195). You can also support your health by eating well (see pp208–249).

All these elements come together in yoga. In fact, the Sanskrit word yoga means "union." Practicing yoga helps the body to find its natural balance and teaches the mind to be a responsible and intelligent driver of the body.

The five elements

Traditional yogic texts describe the body as a "food sheath" (*anayamaya kosha*), made up of five elements. We maintain health by constantly adjusting the body to bring it into harmony with these five elements.

Earth Bones, muscles, and skin contain this element. Asanas move the earth element in all possible directions.

Water Mainly relates to blood. Asanas improve circulation, balance blood pressure, and strengthen the heart.

Fire Seen in the 97–102°F (36–39°C) range of internal temperatures that the body can survive. Practicing yoga adapts the body to climatic change.

Air Yoga improves the circulation of air in the body. Breathing exercises increase the exchange of gases in the lungs, while asanas boost blood circulation, ensuring proper oxygen and carbon dioxide levels in every cell.

Ether, or space This is the almost empty space at the core of matter, as described by quantum physics. It is here that prana—invisible vital energy—circulates. Yoga postures allow prana to flow freely and breathing exercises increase its vibratory level.

Benefits for the heart

Modern science is now discovering the many health benefits that classical yoga postures bring to mind and body. Among the most important benefits discovered so far is the effect of yoga on the heart.

All physical exercise promotes better blood circulation and a stronger heart. Although yoga is gentler than most other types of exercise, it still provides a good cardiac workout. In addition, when you practice inverted poses, such as Headstand (see pp62–75) or Shoulderstand (see pp76–79), your heart benefits from a unique form of stimulation.

In these inverted, or upside-down, poses, the pull of gravity draws the blood from the legs and lower trunk back to the heart. This boosted blood flow stretches the heart muscle, which then contracts more powerfully, pumping an increased amount of blood to the whole body. However, before you attempt the inverted poses in this book, do read the cautions on pages 62 and 76.

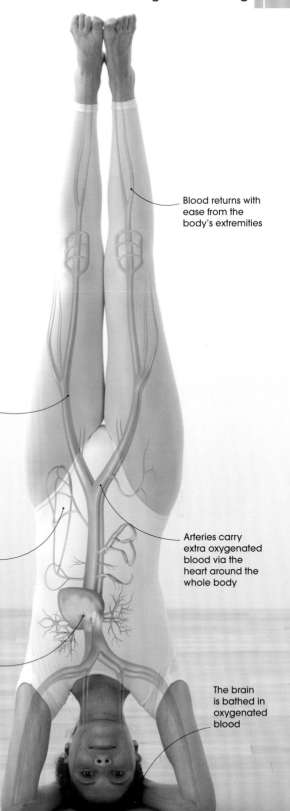

Blood returns with ease from the body's extremities

Veins return more deoxygenated blood to the heart, from where it returns to the lungs

Extra blood reaches every cell in the body, reviving and restoring them

Arteries carry extra oxygenated blood via the heart around the whole body

Stretched by the boosted blood flow, the heart contracts more powerfully

The brain is bathed in oxygenated blood

INVERSIONS FOR HEALTH
In inverted poses, such as **Headstand**, there is increased blood flow back to the heart. This gives you an effortless cardiac workout.

Muscles and movement

Asanas promote health by increasing the range of motion in the joints, keeping the body mobile. At most joints, muscles are arranged in opposing pairs: movement takes place when one muscle contracts, or shortens, while the other relaxes and lengthens.

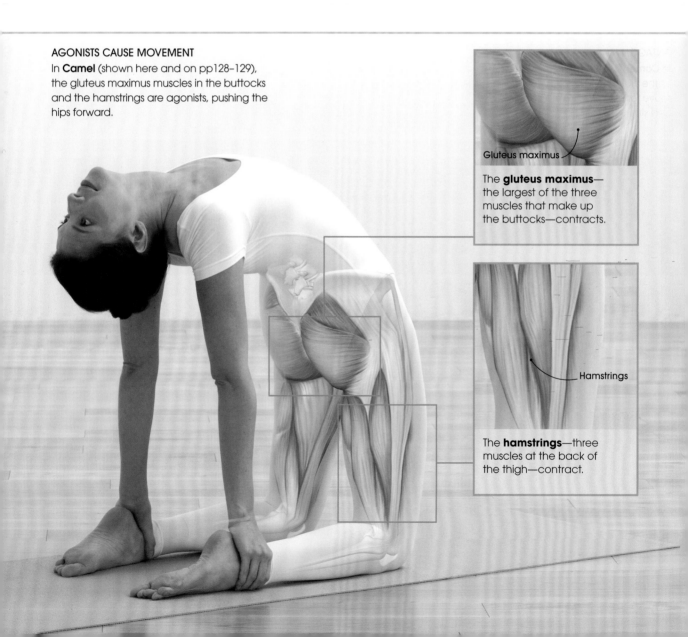

AGONISTS CAUSE MOVEMENT
In **Camel** (shown here and on pp128–129), the gluteus maximus muscles in the buttocks and the hamstrings are agonists, pushing the hips forward.

Gluteus maximus

The **gluteus maximus**—the largest of the three muscles that make up the buttocks—contracts.

Hamstrings

The **hamstrings**—three muscles at the back of the thigh—contract.

Contraction and relaxation

AGONIST MUSCLES A muscle is called an "agonist" when its contraction causes movement in a joint. For example, in Camel, the contraction of the gluteus maximus acts as an agonist, causing the movement of the thigh in the hip joint. If the gluteus maximus is not strong enough to contract fully, you will lack full range of movement in the hip joint.

ANTAGONIST MUSCLES A muscle is an "antagonist" when its role in a movement is to relax, or stretch. In Camel, the iliopsoas (hip-flexor muscles) act as antagonists. If they do not stretch enough, even if the agonist (e.g. gluteus maximus) contracts strongly, you will not succeed in having a completely mobile hip joint.

ANTAGONISTS RELAX
In **Camel**, the strong iliopsoas muscles at the hips work as antagonists: the hips move forward only if these can relax and stretch.

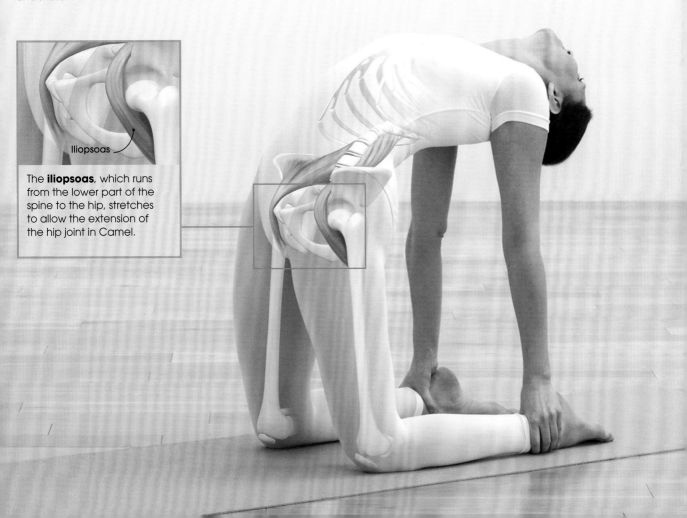

Iliopsoas

The **iliopsoas**, which runs from the lower part of the spine to the hip, stretches to allow the extension of the hip joint in Camel.

ISOMETRIC CONTRACTION Usually, a muscle shortens when it contracts. But in this form of movement, a muscle contracts without shortening. For example, in the Triangle with Bent Knee (see below and p168) variation, the quadriceps (front thigh muscle) of the bent leg contracts strongly. In most cases, this would extend the knee and straighten the leg, but with isometric contraction, the knee remains bent while the thigh muscles contract strongly in order to resist the pull of gravity.

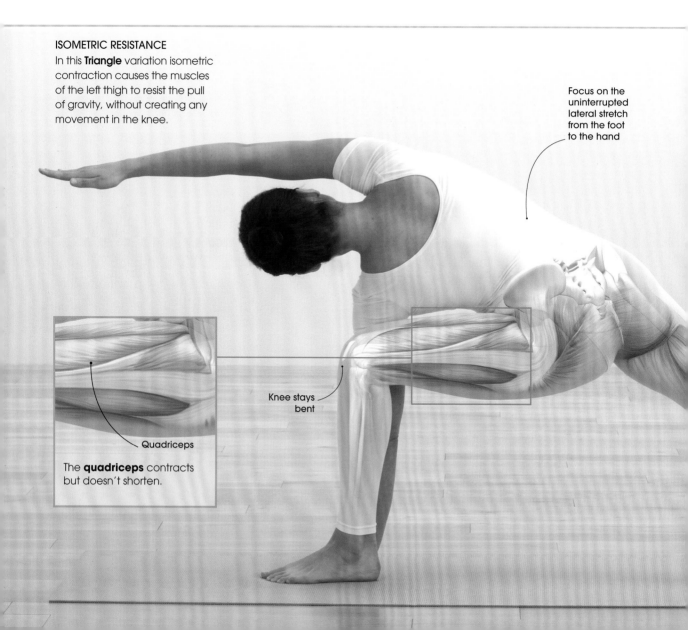

ISOMETRIC RESISTANCE

In this **Triangle** variation isometric contraction causes the muscles of the left thigh to resist the pull of gravity, without creating any movement in the knee.

Focus on the uninterrupted lateral stretch from the foot to the hand

Knee stays bent

Quadriceps

The **quadriceps** contracts but doesn't shorten.

ISOTONIC CONTRACTION In this form of muscle contraction, a muscle shortens, causing a movement in the joint. For example, in Shoulderstand (shown here and on p78), the biceps contract, causing the elbows to bend. This is the most common form of muscle contraction

ISOTONIC FLEXION In **Shoulderstand**, an isotonic contraction of the biceps muscles in the upper arms creates a flexion, or bend, in the elbows. This allows you to push your torso and legs up into the inverted position.

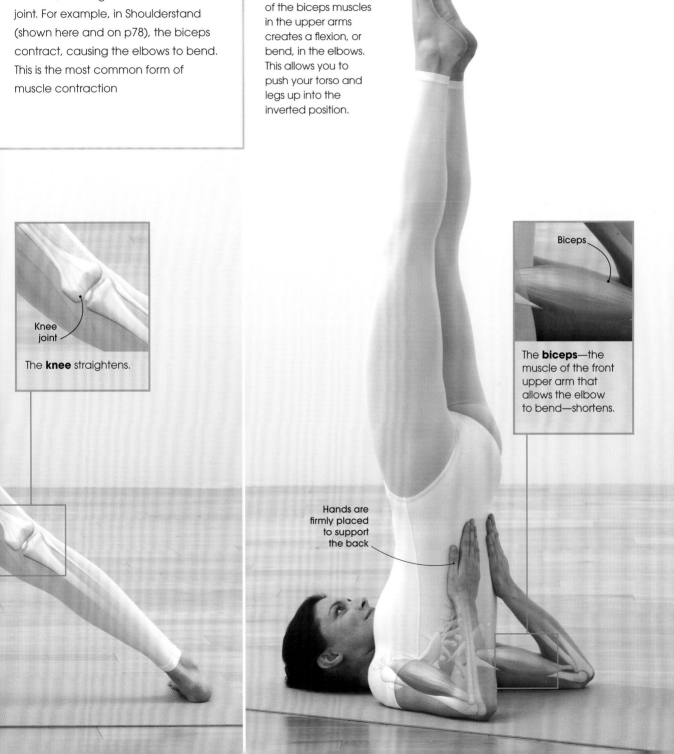

Knee joint

The **knee** straightens.

Biceps

The **biceps**—the muscle of the front upper arm that allows the elbow to bend—shortens.

Hands are firmly placed to support the back

ECCENTRIC CONTRACTION This form of muscular contraction occurs when a muscle contracts and stretches at the same time. In the basic Triangle (shown here and p165), the lateral (sideways) flexion of the spine creates a deep stretch in the iliopsoas muscles in the pelvis. At the same time, the trunk is held parallel to the floor and the lower

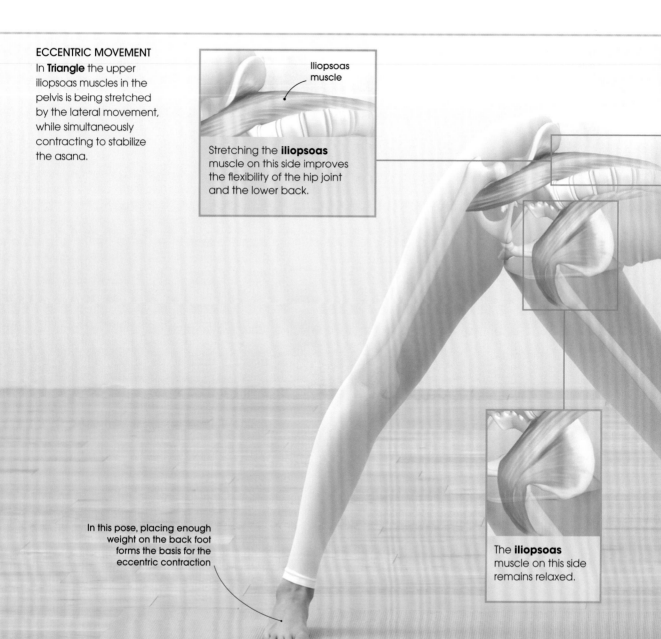

ECCENTRIC MOVEMENT
In **Triangle** the upper iliopsoas muscles in the pelvis is being stretched by the lateral movement, while simultaneously contracting to stabilize the asana.

Iliopsoas muscle

Stretching the **iliopsoas** muscle on this side improves the flexibility of the hip joint and the lower back.

In this pose, placing enough weight on the back foot forms the basis for the eccentric contraction

The **iliopsoas** muscle on this side remains relaxed.

arm is not allowed to support the body weight. This forces the iliopsoas muscle fibers to contract as they are stretching.

Proper eccentric contraction requires good body awareness, which is one reason why Triangle and its variations are practiced at the end of a yoga session.

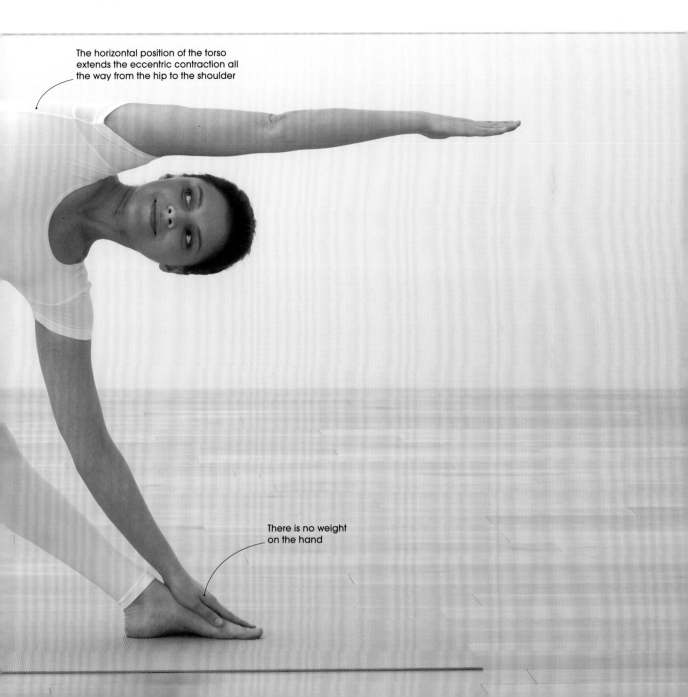

The horizontal position of the torso extends the eccentric contraction all the way from the hip to the shoulder

There is no weight on the hand

STRETCHING FROM FOOT TO HEAD Muscles do not only cause or prevent movement in specific joints (see agonist and antagonist, pp20–21). They can also be arranged in long chains, which transmit either a muscle stretch or a muscle contraction from one end of the body to the other. These chains are created by a special form of connective tissue called

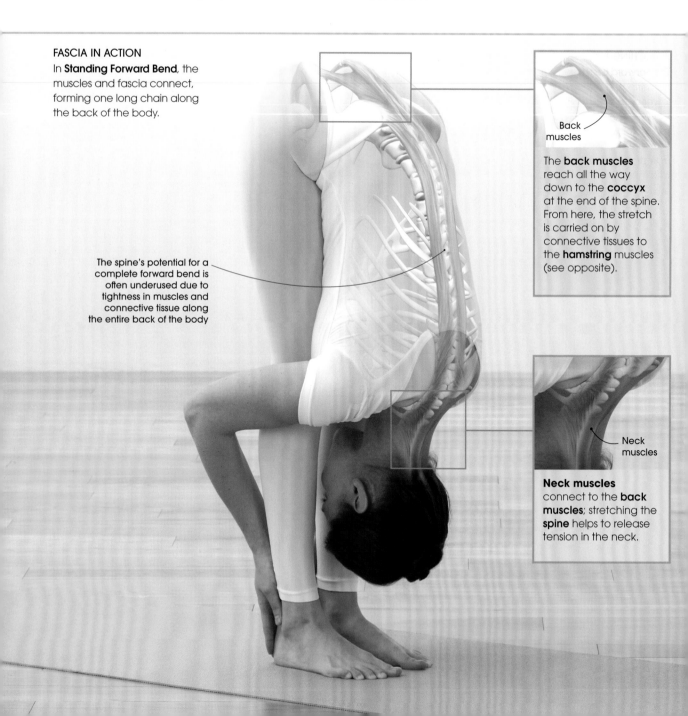

FASCIA IN ACTION
In **Standing Forward Bend**, the muscles and fascia connect, forming one long chain along the back of the body.

The spine's potential for a complete forward bend is often underused due to tightness in muscles and connective tissue along the entire back of the body

Back muscles

The **back muscles** reach all the way down to the **coccyx** at the end of the spine. From here, the stretch is carried on by connective tissues to the **hamstring** muscles (see opposite).

Neck muscles

Neck muscles connect to the **back muscles**; stretching the **spine** helps to release tension in the neck.

"fascia." Fascia surrounds every muscle cell and each muscle as a whole. It also connects one muscle with another. Fascia is what allows the powerful, complete stretch along the back of the body in Standing Forward Bend shown here (see also p163). For additional information on connective tissue, see p28.

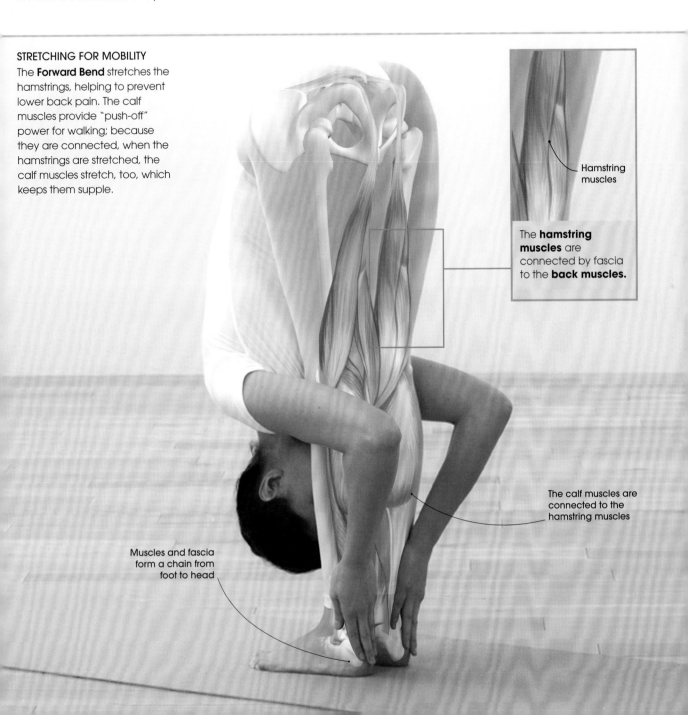

STRETCHING FOR MOBILITY

The **Forward Bend** stretches the hamstrings, helping to prevent lower back pain. The calf muscles provide "push-off" power for walking; because they are connected, when the hamstrings are stretched, the calf muscles stretch, too, which keeps them supple.

Hamstring muscles

The **hamstring muscles** are connected by fascia to the **back muscles.**

The calf muscles are connected to the hamstring muscles

Muscles and fascia form a chain from foot to head

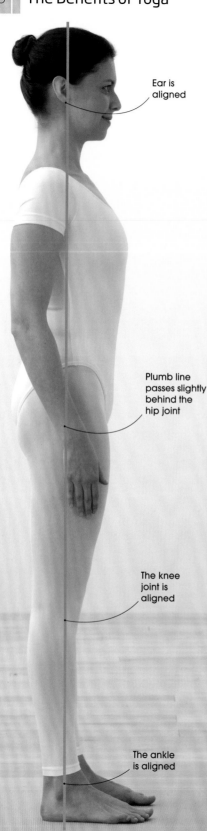

Ear is aligned

Plumb line passes slightly behind the hip joint

The knee joint is aligned

The ankle is aligned

Aligning the posture

Most people don't have well-aligned posture. Practicing asanas focuses on strengthening and stretching key muscles. This will help gradually to improve any faulty alignment, particularly in the upper and lower back.

How the body benefits

Aligning your posture involves improving the balance between muscle length and muscle strength. Yoga does this perfectly, because when you hold an asana and then practice its counterpose, the major muscles on the front and back of the body are both stretched and strengthened. This creates tone as well as flexibility. Yoga asanas also have a positive effect on the muscles' connective tissue, or fascia (see pp26–27). Muscles are elastic: after they stretch or contract, the fibers return to their original length. Fascia, however, is plastic not elastic, which means that only if enough pressure is applied, will it change its form and not revert to its previous shape when the pressure is removed. Constant repetition of certain movements or body positions, such as always carrying a bag on one shoulder or hunching in front of a computer, fixes the connective tissue into a belt-like, non-elastic structure, causing postural problems. When you hold an asana for longer than a minute, this hardened connective tissue starts to be remodeled, bringing your posture back into proper alignment.

GOOD ALIGNMENT
When someone who has correct posture stands beside a plumb line, the ankles, knees, hips, and ears are aligned perfectly, stacked one above the other in a straight line.

Corrective asanas for kyphosis

Kyphosis, or an exaggerated curve of the spine in the upper back, is a common problem of postural alignment, which is exacerbated by slouching or spending long hours hunching forward over a computer. These specific asanas gently help to bring the spine into alignment.

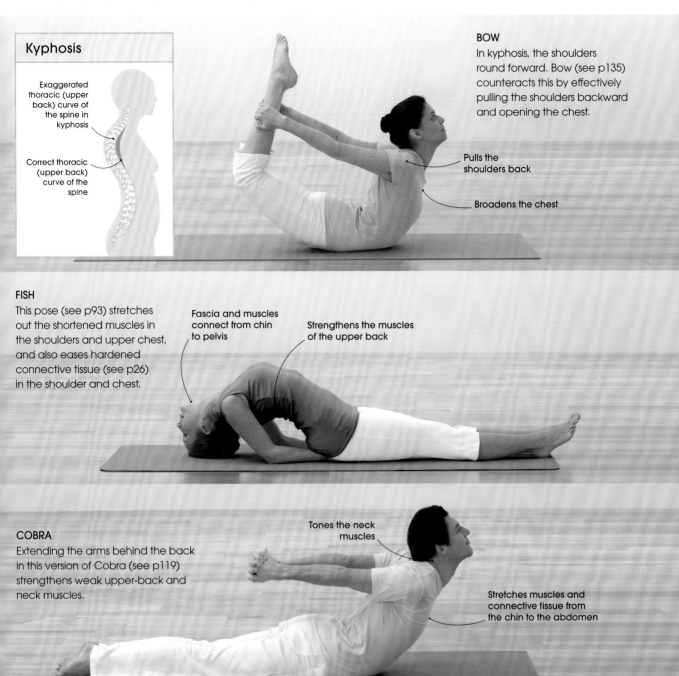

Kyphosis

Exaggerated thoracic (upper back) curve of the spine in kyphosis

Correct thoracic (upper back) curve of the spine

BOW
In kyphosis, the shoulders round forward. Bow (see p135) counteracts this by effectively pulling the shoulders backward and opening the chest.

Pulls the shoulders back

Broadens the chest

FISH
This pose (see p93) stretches out the shortened muscles in the shoulders and upper chest, and also eases hardened connective tissue (see p26) in the shoulder and chest.

Fascia and muscles connect from chin to pelvis

Strengthens the muscles of the upper back

COBRA
Extending the arms behind the back in this version of Cobra (see p119) strengthens weak upper-back and neck muscles.

Tones the neck muscles

Stretches muscles and connective tissue from the chin to the abdomen

Corrective asanas for lordosis

In this condition, the muscles of the abdomen tend to be weak, and the hamstrings and lower back muscles have become shortened. Connective tissue (see pp26–27) along the back of the legs and back has hardened. These poses help to strengthen and lengthen the muscles and soften the tissue.

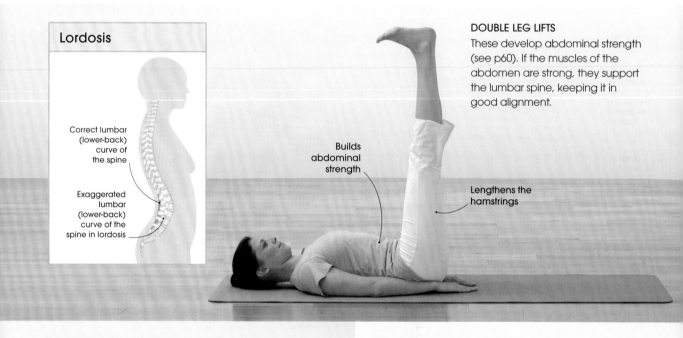

Lordosis

Correct lumbar (lower-back) curve of the spine

Exaggerated lumbar (lower-back) curve of the spine in lordosis

DOUBLE LEG LIFTS
These develop abdominal strength (see p60). If the muscles of the abdomen are strong, they support the lumbar spine, keeping it in good alignment.

Builds abdominal strength

Lengthens the hamstrings

SITTING FORWARD BEND

This pose (see p99) gives a deep stretch to the muscles of the back of the body, which have become shortened. Try to hold the pose for some time, stretching slowly and gradually. As long as any pain that comes from the natural stretch can be dissolved by rhythmical abdominal breathing and relaxation, it is safe to remain in the posture. Any other pain should be taken as a warning sign not to take the stretch too far.

Lengthens the muscles of the lower back

Stretches the hamstrings

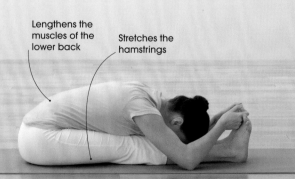

STANDING FORWARD BEND

Another stretch to lengthen the whole of the back of the body (see pp163). As you stretch, use slow, controlled breathing and consciously relax. This, together with repeated practice, will ease any pain and boost flexibility.

Lengthens the lower spine

Stretches the backs of the legs

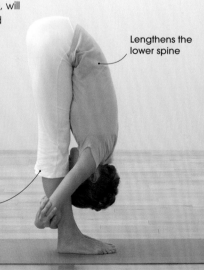

Corrective asanas for scoliosis

When the spinal muscles diagonally opposite each other are shortened on one side and overstretched on the other, it leads to scoliosis. For example, the left side of the lumbar and the right side of the thoracic spine could be pulled out of alignment. Holding asanas to the right and left rebalances the muscles.

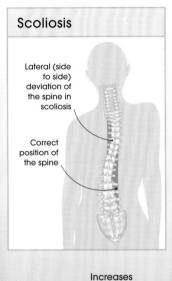

Scoliosis

Lateral (side to side) deviation of the spine in scoliosis

Correct position of the spine

HALF SPINAL TWIST

Hold this pose (see p148)—and all other poses on this page—for the same length of time on each side. This ensures automatic stretching and strengthening in all the required areas.

Increases flexibility on one side

Tones the muscles on the other side

TRIANGLE

Asanas such as Triangle (see p165) that are practiced to the right and left sides restore the correct balance of flexibility and strength to the muscles on either side of the spine. They also help to soften hardened connective tissue, or fascia.

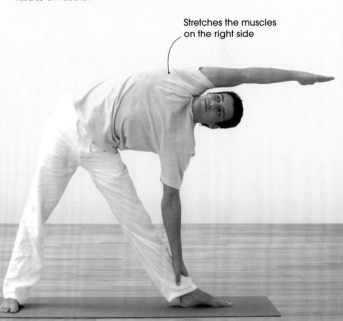

Stretches the muscles on the right side

LATERAL BEND WITH TWIST

Lateral stretches such as Lateral Bend with Twist (see p107) help to restore the balance of shortened muscles on diagonally opposite sides of the spine. Always move slowly into the pose to overcome gradually any inherent resistance in the muscles.

Stretches from hip to shoulder

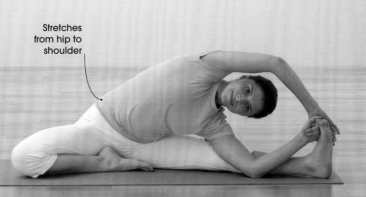

The breath of life

Breathing is like no other body function because it connects us with our environment. Plants take in carbon dioxide and give off oxygen, while human beings and animals inhale oxygen-rich air and exhale air high in carbon dioxide. Yoga breathing exercises help to increase the gas exchange in the lungs and in all the cells of the body.

Involuntary breathing

Most of the time we breathe involuntarily, thanks to respiratory-control centers located in the brain. An average adult respiratory rate varies between 12 and 20 breaths per minute at rest, moving about 1 pint (.5 liter) of air in and out of the lungs—this is the vital capacity. When an adult exercises, the respiratory rate can go up to 35–45 breaths per minute, increasing vital capacity to over 8½ pints (4 liters) of inhaled and exhaled air. Such fast, deep breathing is prompted by a sudden increase in carbon-dioxide waste in the muscles caused by exercising.

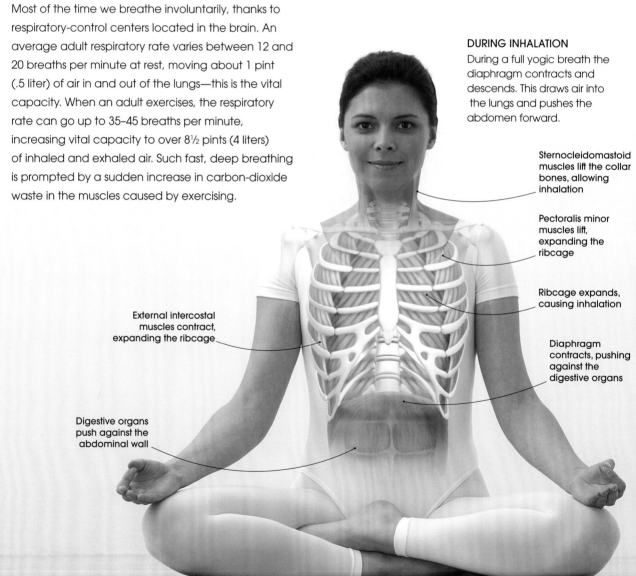

DURING INHALATION
During a full yogic breath the diaphragm contracts and descends. This draws air into the lungs and pushes the abdomen forward.

Sternocleidomastoid muscles lift the collar bones, allowing inhalation

Pectoralis minor muscles lift, expanding the ribcage

Ribcage expands, causing inhalation

Diaphragm contracts, pushing against the digestive organs

External intercostal muscles contract, expanding the ribcage

Digestive organs push against the abdominal wall

Voluntary breath control

Yoga emphasizes voluntary breath control. During asana practice, breathing slows to 10–12 breaths per minute. In relaxation and meditation, you breathe only 6–8 times per minute, and you take just 3–6 breaths per minute during Alternate Nostril Breathing (see pp182–183). All respiratory training in yoga emphasizes complete exhalation in order to eliminate maximum amounts of stale air and allow a deeper inhalation.

In this way, freshly inhaled oxygen-rich air mixes with lesser amounts of stale air than in involuntary breathing, making more oxygen available to nourish every cell. During pranayama, oxygen levels in the blood are higher when you inhale and much lower when you retain your breath. Studies by the Russian medical researcher Dr. Arkadi F. Prokop suggest that exposure to alternating high and low levels of oxygen promotes cell rejuvenation, speeding up the renewal of mitochondria, the microscopic power plants in every cell. Many asanas create pressure on the chest and abdomen. Performing a complete yogic breath (see p180) against such resistance strengthens the respiratory muscles and helps you to breathe with greater awareness in daily life.

DURING EXHALATION
The diaphragm relaxes and moves up, pushing air out of the lungs and allowing the abdomen to move back in.

Sternocleidomastoid muscles relax

Pectoralis minor muscles relax, so the chest drops

External intercostal muscles relax, so the chest sinks

Diaphragm relaxes

Abdominal muscles contract, pushing internal organs against the diaphragm for complete exhalation

Supporting the nervous system

Yoga works on the nervous system, keeping it in balance so that you feel better able to deal with the unavoidable stresses that are part of daily life. The order of the 12 basic poses and the focus on posture, breathing, and relaxation in each asana help the nervous system function, leading to a sense of complete relaxation and rejuvenation.

What is the autonomic nervous system?

The autonomic nervous system fine-tunes the activities of the vital organs of the body, such as the heart, as well as the respiratory, digestive, and endocrine systems (see p37). It also governs homeostasis (see p18).This system functions involuntarily, ensuring that nerves transmit messages between the brain and organs, muscles, and glands, through the central nervous system in the brain and spinal cord. The autonomic nervous system is divided into two: the sympathetic and parasympathetic systems.

THE SYMPATHETIC NERVOUS SYSTEM This branch of the autonomic nervous system sends out nerve impulses, in response to perceived physical or psychological danger, that triggers the release of hormones including adrenaline and noradrenaline. These prepare the body for fighting the danger or fleeing from it (the "fight or flight response") by stimulating an increase in heart rate and blood pressure, diverting blood to the skeletal muscles, and slowing the digestion and kidney function, among other reactions. These stress responses continue until the body fights or runs away or the parasympathetic nervous system becomes dominant. If the responses are not dispelled, over time they can damage the body and mind.

THE PARASYMPATHETIC NERVOUS SYSTEM The other branch of the autonomic nervous system promotes rest, energy conservation, and the absorption of nutrients to maintain good health. It also supports the regular functioning of the cardiovascular, digestive, and excretory systems among other vital processes, and acts as an antidote to the "fight or flight response." Practicing yoga asanas (see pp42–169), pranayama (see pp176–185), and meditation (see pp196–207) activates this "rest and repair" branch of the autonomic nervous system.

Sympathetic and parasympathetic activity

The two systems work in a complementary way. As the brain anticipates danger, the sympathetic neurons in the spinal cord release chemical nerve transmitters. These trigger target organs, muscles, and glands to prepare to deal with stress by reacting as shown below. When the parasympathetic nerves are stimulated, they gradually undo these responses.

PARASYMPATHETIC SYSTEM   SYMPATHETIC SYSTEM

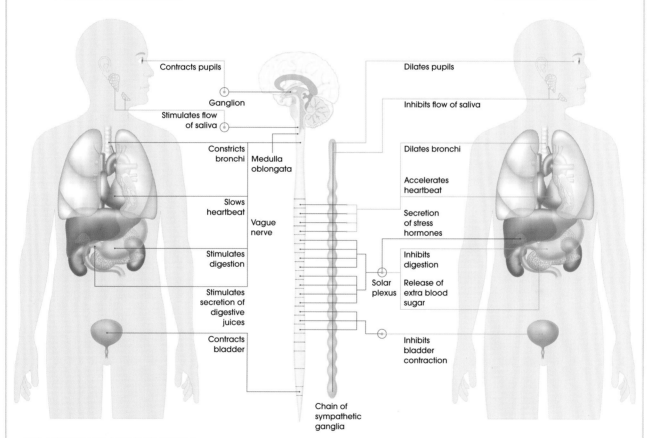

Contracts pupils

Ganglion

Stimulates flow of saliva

Constricts bronchi | Medulla oblongata

Slows heartbeat

Vague nerve

Stimulates digestion

Stimulates secretion of digestive juices

Contracts bladder

Chain of sympathetic ganglia

Dilates pupils

Inhibits flow of saliva

Dilates bronchi

Accelerates heartbeat

Secretion of stress hormones

Solar plexus | Inhibits digestion

Release of extra blood sugar

Inhibits bladder contraction

THE AUTONOMIC NERVOUS SYSTEM

The sympathetic system is important because it primes us to deal with stressful situations, promoting alertness and quick-thinking. When the parasympathetic system is in action after a period of sympathetic activity, it provides optimum conditions for good health.

Yoga to balance the nervous system

Structuring your asana practice in the following way can help to restore the balance between the sympathetic and parasympathetic nervous systems.

SUN SALUTATION At the beginning of your asana session, practice Sun Salutations (see pp50–57), to start reducing sympathetic nerve impulses.

ALTERNATE MUSCLE STRETCHING AND RELAXATION Then practice asanas that focus mostly on flexibility (see pp58–115), following them with an appropriate relaxation pose. Alternating the slight muscle pain of stretching with relaxation stimulates the parasympathetic nervous system, helping you to relax.

ALTERNATING MUSCLE CONTRACTION AND RELAXATION Now you will do mostly short, intense muscle contractions (see pp116–169) followed by conscious relaxation to prompt the "rest and repair" impulses in the parasympathetic system.

FINAL RELAXATION During final relaxation (see pp192–193), your body is flooded with parasympathetic nerve impulses. When you return to a stressful situation your sympathetic nerve impulses may be stimulated again, but thanks to the strength of the parasympathetic "rest and repair" impulses you experience in your asana practice, they will have little effect on you.

Muscle stretching and relaxation

Notice how any pain you feel in the muscles during the stretches disappears completely during the complementary relaxation pose. You are literally stretching the stress away.

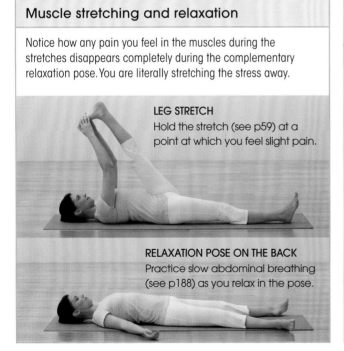

LEG STRETCH
Hold the stretch (see p59) at a point at which you feel slight pain.

RELAXATION POSE ON THE BACK
Practice slow abdominal breathing (see p188) as you relax in the pose.

Muscle contraction and relaxation

Some asanas demand more dynamic muscle work. When followed immediately by an appropriate relaxation pose, you stimulate the parasympathetic nervous system.

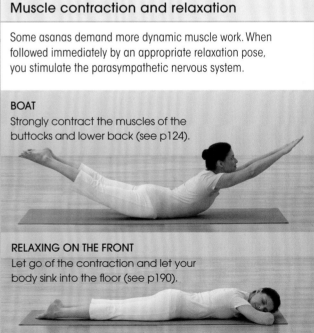

BOAT
Strongly contract the muscles of the buttocks and lower back (see p124).

RELAXING ON THE FRONT
Let go of the contraction and let your body sink into the floor (see p190).

Yoga and the endocrine system

The endocrine glands secrete hormones into the blood stream. These chemical "messengers" reach every cell of the body. They initiate and regulate many body functions. Yoga helps to keep this body system in good shape.

What does it do?

The main endocrine gland is the pituitary gland in the brain. Other glands include the pineal, also in the brain, which produces melatonin to control the sleep-wake cycle, and the thyroid in the neck, which releases hormones regulating growth and metabolism. At the back of this gland is the parathyroid, which promotes calcium absorption. The thymus at the top of the chest regulates immunity; the adrenals on top of each kidney oversee fluid balance, fat distribution, and stress hormones. The pancreas, an organ, regulates blood-sugar levels and the ovaries or testes release sex hormones.

Benefits for the brain

Practicing asanas helps to bring balance to the brain and, through the pituitary gland, to the whole body. In certain asanas, such as Headstand, extra blood circulates to the brain, nourishing it with oxygen and nutrients. This improves the working of the hypothalamus.

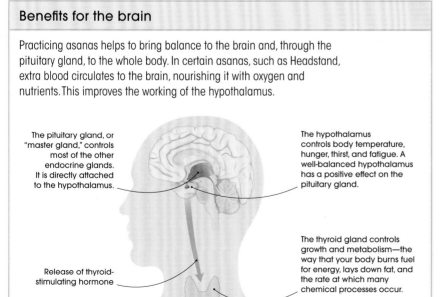

The pituitary gland, or "master gland," controls most of the other endocrine glands. It is directly attached to the hypothalamus.

The hypothalamus controls body temperature, hunger, thirst, and fatigue. A well-balanced hypothalamus has a positive effect on the pituitary gland.

Release of thyroid-stimulating hormone

The thyroid gland controls growth and metabolism—the way that your body burns fuel for energy, lays down fat, and the rate at which many chemical processes occur.

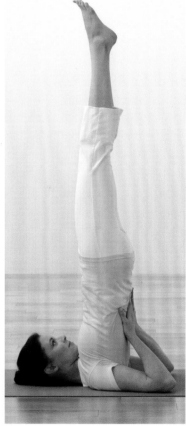

SHOULDERSTAND
When you hold this pose (see p78), you increase the blood circulation in the thyroid gland in the neck, which promotes a healthy metabolism.

Yoga and relaxation

Yoga teaches you how to achieve deep muscle relaxation, first by following a muscle contraction in one asana with complete muscular relaxation in its complementary resting pose. Second, by using autosuggestion in final relaxation (see pp192–194), asking each part of the body in turn to relax until you experience a feeling of total release.

A strong muscle contraction requires an intense number of nerve impulses to command muscle fibers to shorten; complete relaxation requires the fewest nerve impulses to be directed to the fibers. These processes seem opposed, but the more you relax before moving into an asana, the more efficiently you will be able to focus on muscle contraction, and the deeper you will be able to breathe. Follow the asana with its relaxation pose; then the complete release of the contraction plus slow breathing stimulates deep relaxation.

Using autosuggestion

To achieve deep muscle relaxation in final relaxation (see pp192–194), lie comfortably, then create a mental picture of the muscles of the body in turn, and send them a mental command to relax, which travels via impulses from the motor cortex in the brain. The command is followed quickly by a feeling of relaxation.

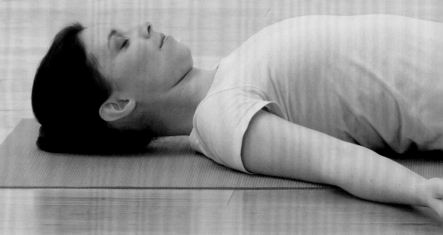

COMPLETE RELAXATION
Working from your feet to your head, you can use step-by-step muscle relaxation with autosuggestion to achieve a sense of deep relaxation.

Location of cortexes

The motor cortex and the somatic sensory cortex sit alongside each other in the brain.

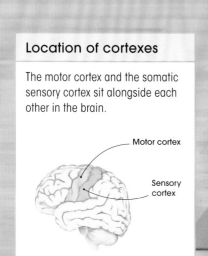

Motor cortex

Sensory cortex

Brain mapping

This "map" of the motor cortex and the somatic sensory cortex (see location, opposite) shows the relationship between the two. Since they are so close to each other, when you ask a specific part of the body to relax, an impulse travels from the relevant area of the sensory cortex with a message to the motor cortex and the body part immediately feels relaxed.

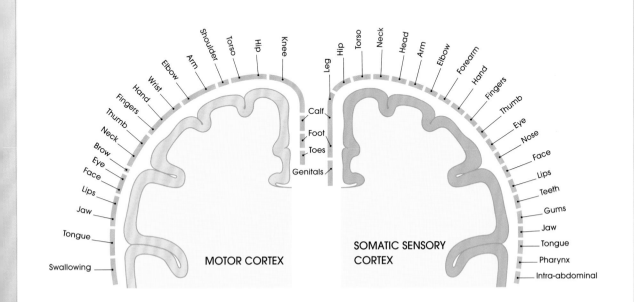

MOTOR CORTEX

SOMATIC SENSORY CORTEX

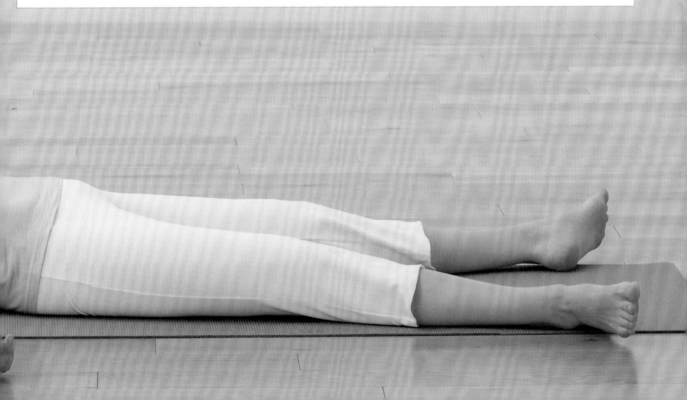

One pose, many benefits

Asanas work on many body systems simultaneously. Gaining a better understanding of how some of these benefits complement each other can bring you one step closer to understanding the Sanskrit word yoga, which translates as "union." Here, we look at the benefits a single asana can bring to many parts of the body and the mind.

Effects on the body

Practicing this variation of Triangle pose (see p167) benefits all ten body systems, from the skeletal to the reproductive, but these in particular:

MUSCULAR SYSTEM The muscles at the front of the thighs contract to keep the leg stable, while those at the back of the thighs extend. Balancing muscle strength with length maintains mobility in the joints. Repeating the pose to both sides promotes good posture by working the spine evenly.

NERVOUS SYSTEM The spine, containing the central nervous system, receives a good stretch along its length, which benefits communication between the spinal nerves and the brain. The cerebellum controls smooth movement, proper alignment, and stable posture.

ENDOCRINE SYSTEM Blood flows easily to the brain in this pose, supporting the pituitary gland (see p37), which regulates hormone secretion throughout the body. More specifically, the pressure of the pose stimulates the adrenal gland. This helps to ensure its role in the "fight or flight response" (see p34) and in processing food and regulating energy.

DIGESTIVE SYSTEM As the trunk revolves, the digestive organs receive a massage, which stimulates the functioning of the digestive system. The pressure on the organs pushes stagnating blood out of them, which in turn draws fresh blood supply into this area, once the pose is released.

CARDIOVASCULAR AND RESPIRATORY SYSTEMS This pose requires some exertion, working the muscles of the heart and increasing the lungs' vital capacity (see p32–33). The respiratory muscles also get a good workout from working against the compression of the twist. Both actions ensure a good supply of oxygen to the brain, encouraging concentration and vitality.

What happens in the brain

The pose activates the cerebellum to maintain balance. It also massages the adrenal glands on top of the kidneys, whose function is controlled by the pituitary gland in the brain.

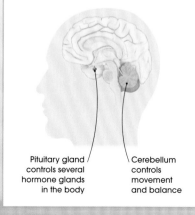

Pituitary gland controls several hormone glands in the body

Cerebellum controls movement and balance

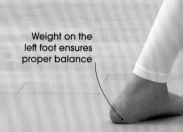

Weight on the left foot ensures proper balance

Massage of the digestive system makes it work more efficiently

Massage of the adrenal glands helps deal with stress

Rotation of the spine tones the spinal nerves and improves their communication with the brain

Eccentric muscle contraction on the left side of the back keeps the torso aligned horizontally

The left hip rotates inward

The cerebellum is stimulated into controlling balance

The right hip rotates outward

The pituitary gland controls the secretions of the adrenal gland

The hamstring muscles of the right leg stretch deeply

TRIANGLE POSE
As well as the benefits on the various body systems, this asana enhances balance and spatial awareness.

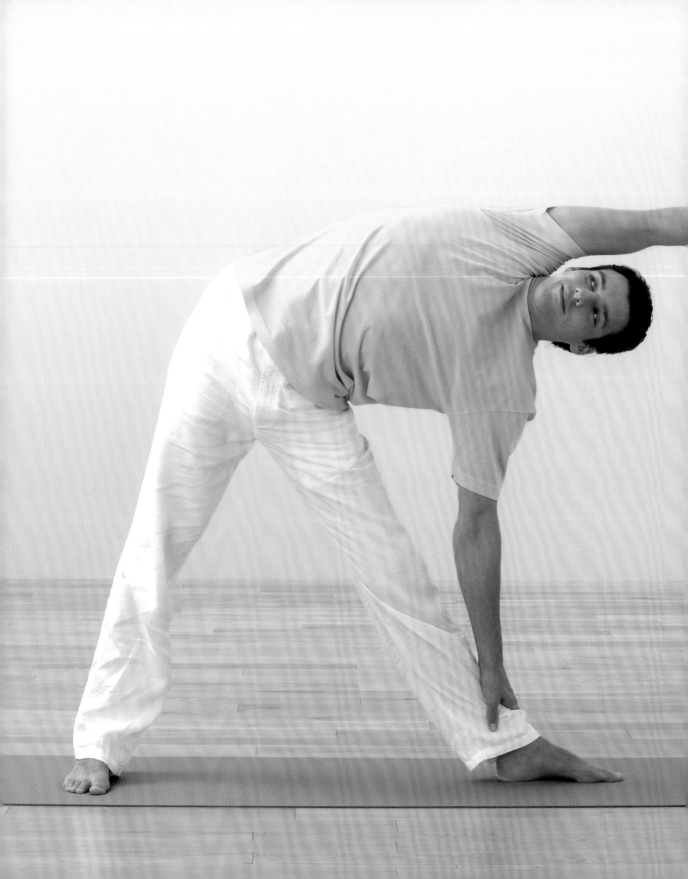

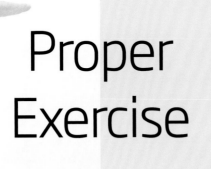

Proper
Exercise

What is proper exercise?

The twelve basic postures, or asanas, should be practiced in a specific order. The aim is to promote good health and to awaken the subtle energy—prana (see p178)—in your body. After you have finished your yoga practice, you will feel a profound sense of physical and emotional well-being.

A logical sequence

The sequence of twelve basic asanas are specially designed to help your body and mind to reap the greatest possible benefits. They should be followed in the order given in this book and you should practice them at every session. Also take care to follow any breathing instructions given, as well as the guidelines for relaxation poses in between asanas.

INITIAL RELAXATION Always begin with relaxation in Corpse Pose (see p46) to focus your mind and prevent you from being distracted by the demands of everyday life. Continue with Easy Sitting Pose (see p47). This gives you a firm sitting position for performing the Eye and Neck Exercises (see pp48–49), as well as the breathing exercises (see pp180-185). Next comes the Sun Salutation (see pp50–57), which stimulates the heart and the circulation of the blood. It also serves as a general warm-up for the poses that follow.

THE FIRST HALF OF YOUR PRACTICE After the Sun Salutation, you move on to asanas that focus mostly on muscle stretching. The stretching is always followed by relaxation of the muscles. In addition, the inverted poses of this first part of your practice increase the blood supply to the head, which improves the function of the brain and thyroid gland.

THE SECOND HALF OF YOUR PRACTICE From Cobra onward (see p116), the asanas focus more on muscle strengthening. This is done by contracting then relaxing the muscles. In addition, poses such as Bow (see pp134–143), Half Spinal Twist (pp144–149), and Peacock (see pp154–161), exert more pressure on your inner organs. This helps to detoxify the tissues and increase their blood supply.

FINAL RELAXATION Practice final relaxation lying in Corpse Pose (see pp192–193). Never omit this essential part of your practice. When you relax in this position, your voluntary muscles and your internal organs relax completely. Final relaxation also helps you to absorb all the benefits of the asanas you have just practiced.

When to practice

You can schedule your yoga practice anytime from early morning to late evening. The most important considerations are:

- You should not eat 2–3 hours before you practice.

- Except late in the evening, you should have a wholesome meal or snack shortly after you practice.

- Taking a shower before you practice is advantageous, but a shower is not recommended immediately after, as it neutralizes prana (see p178).

- Choose a time when you will not be distracted by phone calls.

From beginner to advanced

The step-by-step instructions in this book guide you from beginner level, through intermediate to advanced. If you are a beginner, you may find that, to start with, you can only manage a few of the steps leading up to the final pose. If this is the case, do not worry and do not force yourself on to the next step. It is not a competition. In yoga, there are benefits for mind and body at every step. When you reach the final pose, look at the illustration showing the common faults in the pose. You may be doing some or all of these. As you practice the pose, try and be aware of your mistakes and do your best to correct them.

Pose and counterpose

Many poses have a counterpose—one that moves the spine and other joints in the opposite direction. So, having performed Shoulderstand (see pp76–78), which gives you a forward bend, Fish (see pp92–93), which is another basic asana in its own right, provides you with a backward bend a little later on in your practice.

Clothing and equipment

Loose cotton clothing that enables you to move easily is ideal. You will also need a rubber mat for practicing asanas, and a pillow when you practice the easy sitting position (see p47). You may also like to cover yourself with a thin blanket during final relaxation (see pp192–193).

THE ASANAS AND THEIR VARIATIONS
Most of the twelve basic asanas also have variations. Some variations are poses in their own right, such as Wheel (see pp140–143). Other variations lead on from the basic pose, but take you into more advanced positions, such as this Shoulderstand variation, Arms on Floor (see p79).

Initial Relaxation

Each step of your yoga session demands a fine-tuning of your nervous system. That is why you should always prepare yourself for your asana practice with at least five minutes of complete

Corpse Pose

Lie flat on your back with your arms and legs apart and your eyes closed. Shake out your shoulders to release any tension in them. Slowly roll your head from side to side a couple of times, lowering one ear toward the ground, then the other. Bring your head back to the center. Lie still as you concentrate on your breath, using the deep abdominal breathing technique described below.

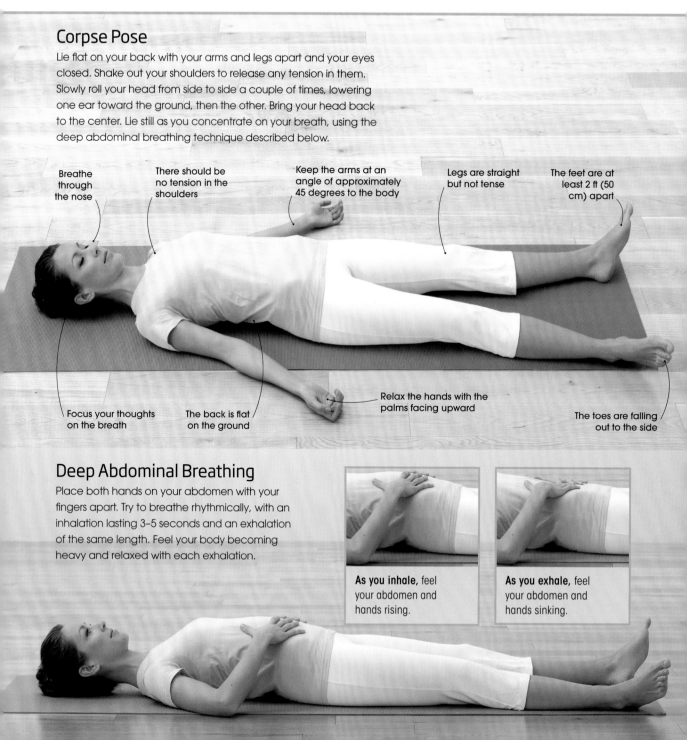

Breathe through the nose

There should be no tension in the shoulders

Keep the arms at an angle of approximately 45 degrees to the body

Legs are straight but not tense

The feet are at least 2 ft (50 cm) apart

Focus your thoughts on the breath

The back is flat on the ground

Relax the hands with the palms facing upward

The toes are falling out to the side

Deep Abdominal Breathing

Place both hands on your abdomen with your fingers apart. Try to breathe rhythmically, with an inhalation lasting 3–5 seconds and an exhalation of the same length. Feel your body becoming heavy and relaxed with each exhalation.

As you inhale, feel your abdomen and hands rising.

As you exhale, feel your abdomen and hands sinking.

relaxation in Corpse Pose, using Deep Abdominal Breathing. Following that, sit in Easy Sitting Pose for 2 minutes, in readiness for the Eye and Neck Exercises (see pp48–49).

Easy Sitting Pose

Sit in a simple, cross-legged position to prepare for the Eye and Neck exercises. This position gives you a very firm, stable base and helps to keep your energy centered.

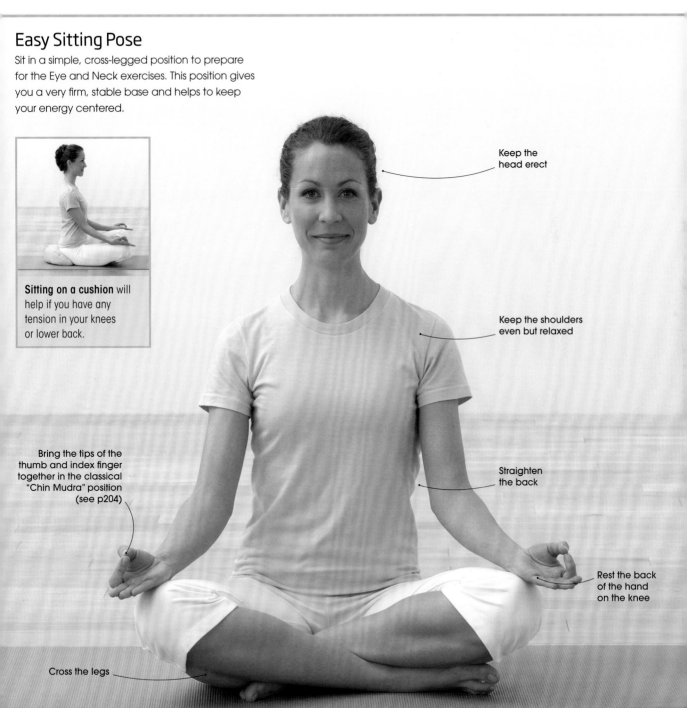

Sitting on a cushion will help if you have any tension in your knees or lower back.

Keep the head erect

Keep the shoulders even but relaxed

Bring the tips of the thumb and index finger together in the classical "Chin Mudra" position (see p204)

Straighten the back

Rest the back of the hand on the knee

Cross the legs

Eye Exercises

In our modern world, the eyes are subjected daily to computer and TV screens, fast-moving traffic, and artificial light. Yogic eye exercises are both relaxing and strengthening for the eyes.

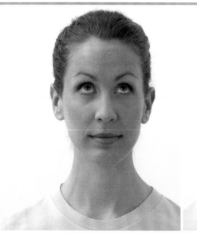 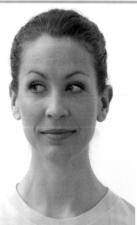 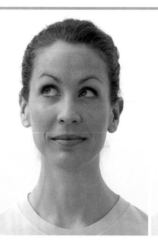 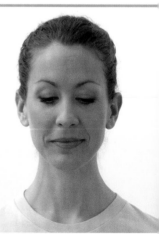

1 Keeping your back and neck straight and your head still, look upward as high as you can, and then look downward. Repeat at least 10 times, then close and relax your eyes for about 30 seconds.

2 Opening your eyes wide, look as far to the right as you can, and then look to the left. Repeat at least 10 times, then close and relax your eyes for 30 seconds.

3 Move your eyes diagonally by looking from the upper right-hand corner to the lower left and back again. Repeat 10 times, then repeat the exercise by looking from the top left corner to the bottom right. Close and relax the eyes.

4 Roll your eyes clockwise in wide circles. Start slowly and gradually increase speed until you are moving your eyes as fast as you can. Make at least 10 circles, then close your eyes for a moment. Now repeat counter-clockwise. Close and relax your eyes.

Relaxing the eyes

To soothe and relax your eyes after the exercises, use warm hands cupped over your eyes to provide heat and darkness.

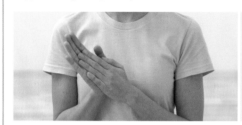 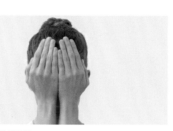

WARMING THE HANDS
When you have finished the eye exercises, rub your hands together vigorously until the friction between them warms up your palms.

CUPPING THE EYES
Gently cup your hands over your closed eyes, without touching the eyelids. Keep them there for about 30 seconds.

Neck Exercises

These exercises aim to release any tension in the neck, shoulders, and upper back. While performing these exercises, only move your head and neck, not your back and shoulders.

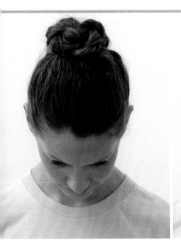

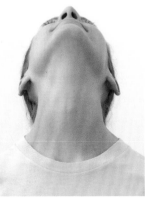

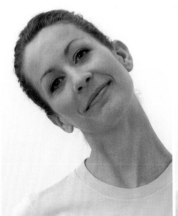

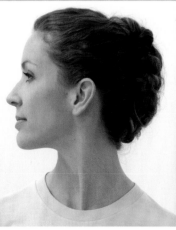

1 Start in the Easy Sitting Position, with your back straight and your chest erect. Slowly bring your head forward toward the chest to give the back of your neck a good stretch.

2 After a few moments slowly lift your head and extend your neck as far back as possible.

3 Lower your right ear close to your right shoulder, then repeat on the opposite side. Keep both shoulders level throughout. Repeat the exercise 5–10 times.

4 Turn your head to the right side. Contract the muscles on the right side of your neck, and feel the stretch on the left side. Repeat on the opposite side. Repeat the exercise 5–10 times.

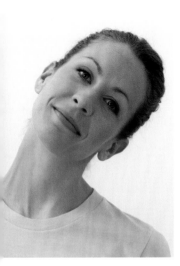

5 Drop your chin to your chest and rotate your head clockwise 2–3 times. Bring your head to the center and start again, performing 2–3 times in a counter-clockwise direction.

CAUTION Some people cannot extend their neck far. If you feel any dizziness or too much pressure on your neck, extend less until you feel comfortable. Repeat the exercise 5-10 times.

Sun Salutation

All Levels

At the start of Sun Salutation, you need to be standing at the front of your mat. This leaves room behind you for the subsequent steps. Observe how the movements involve counter-stretches—

At a glance

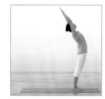 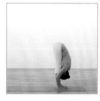 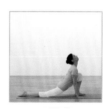 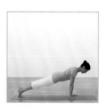 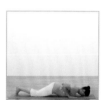

Benefits

PHYSICAL

• Gently increases the blood circulation.

• Thoroughly recharges the solar plexus despite being a physical workout.

• Stretches and strengthens dozens of muscles throughout the body.

• Quickly brings flexibility to the spine and the limbs.

• Regulates the breathing.

• Increases the respiratory capacity.

MENTAL

• Gives a clear sense of being in one place in the present moment, thanks to its symmetrical, circular sequence of movements.

• Looking up and down into space allows the mind to expand.

• The increased and detailed body awareness brings greater detachment. The body is seen as the vehicle of the mind and the soul.

1 Exhale as you bring your palms together in front of your chest in Prayer Position.

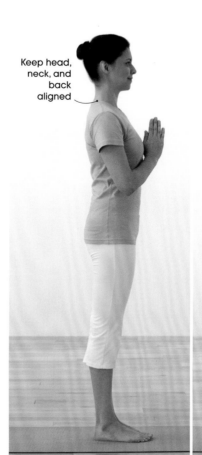

Keep head, neck, and back aligned

Transition to Step 2

Start to inhale as you stretch your arms up next to your ears, palms facing forward. Avoid tension in the neck as you raise your shoulders.

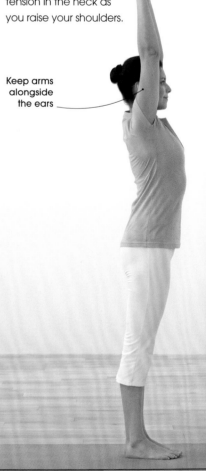

Keep arms alongside the ears

a backward bend followed by a forward bend, which is followed by another backward bend. These movements promote great flexibility in the spine and are beneficial to all levels of practitioner.

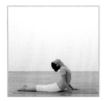 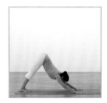 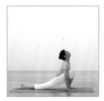 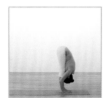 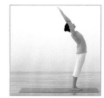 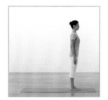

2 As you continue inhaling, take the weight onto your heels, look upward, and arch your arms, head, and chest backward. Stretch your chest and abdomen.

Transition to Step 3

Start to exhale as you bend forward from the waist, keeping your legs straight. Use your back muscles to bring your spine, head, and arms into a horizontal line.

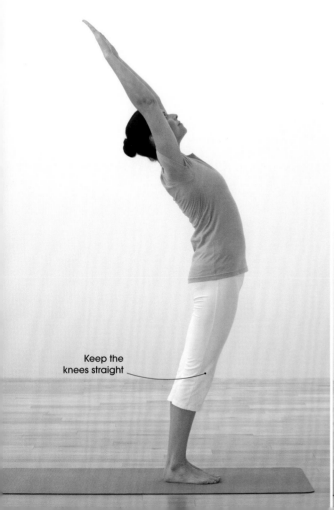

Keep the knees straight

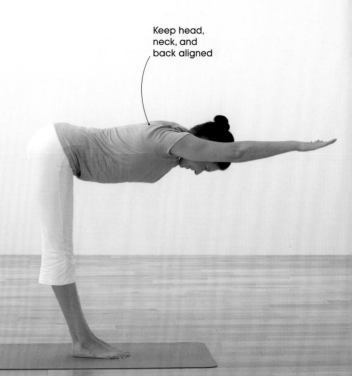

Keep head, neck, and back aligned

Sun Salutation

(continued)

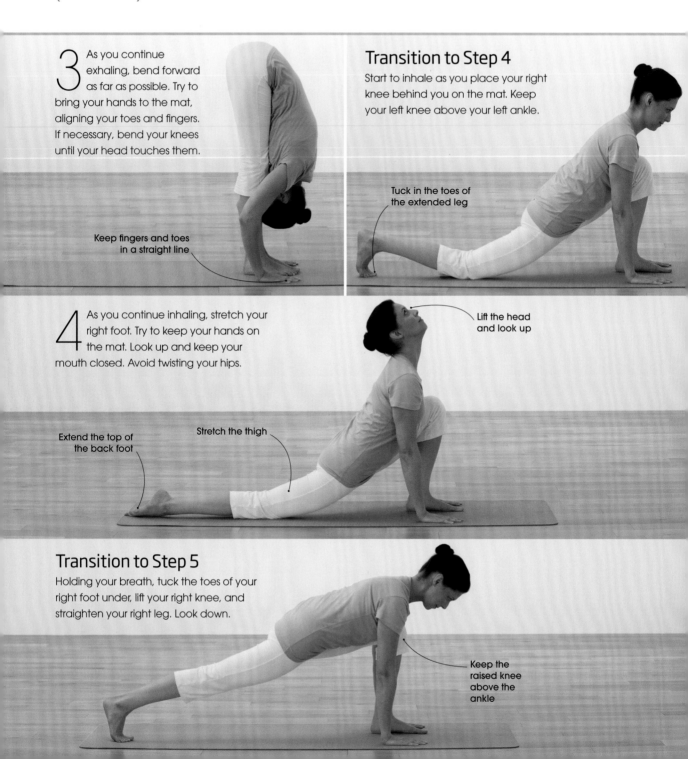

3 As you continue exhaling, bend forward as far as possible. Try to bring your hands to the mat, aligning your toes and fingers. If necessary, bend your knees until your head touches them.

Keep fingers and toes in a straight line

Transition to Step 4

Start to inhale as you place your right knee behind you on the mat. Keep your left knee above your left ankle.

Tuck in the toes of the extended leg

4 As you continue inhaling, stretch your right foot. Try to keep your hands on the mat. Look up and keep your mouth closed. Avoid twisting your hips.

Lift the head and look up

Extend the top of the back foot

Stretch the thigh

Transition to Step 5

Holding your breath, tuck the toes of your right foot under, lift your right knee, and straighten your right leg. Look down.

Keep the raised knee above the ankle

5 Continuing to hold your breath, take your left leg beside your right leg. Align your head, back, hips, and legs. Straighten the legs and look down toward the floor.

Keep the body straight

Transition to Step 6

Start to exhale as you lower your knees to the mat.

Hands remain in position

6 Continuing to exhale, lower your chest and align your shoulders with your fingertips. Take your forehead to the mat, keeping your hips raised.

Keep the hips raised

Place the forehead on the floor

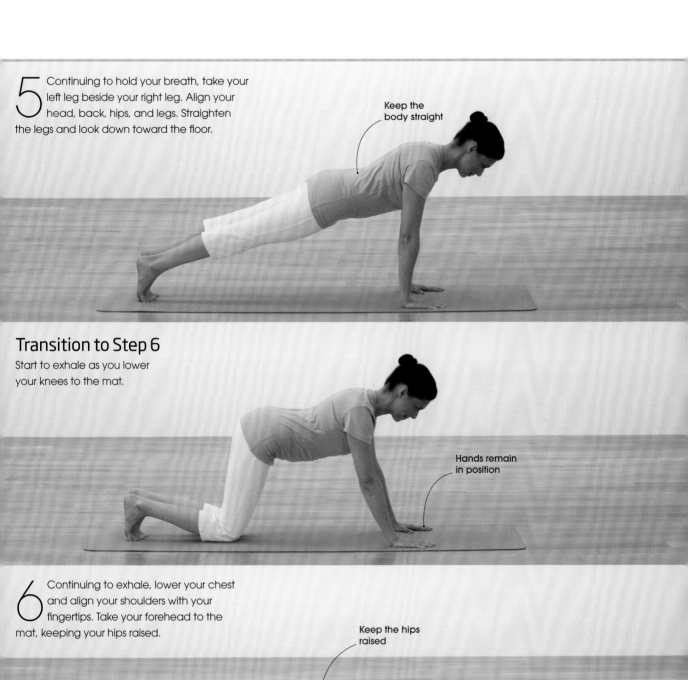

Sun Salutation
(continued)

Transition (a) to Step 7
Start to inhale and, keeping your chest, hands, and forehead in position, lower your hips to the mat. Stretch out your legs and feet.

Head and chest start sliding forward

Transition (b) to Step 7
As you continue inhaling, lift your head and shoulders. Keep your chest on the floor, elbows close to your body, and shoulder blades pulled together. Look up.

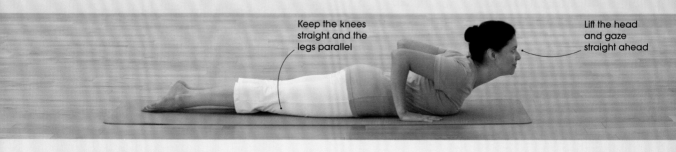

Keep the knees straight and the legs parallel

Lift the head and gaze straight ahead

7 Continue inhaling, arch your head and upper spine backward, keeping your hips on the mat and your shoulders away from your ears. Look up.

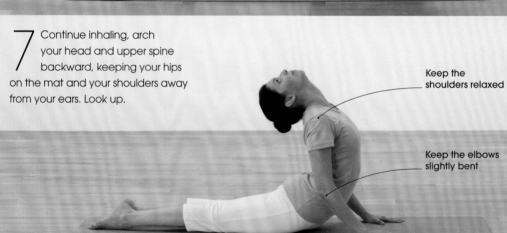

Keep the shoulders relaxed

Keep the elbows slightly bent

Transition to Step 8

Start to exhale as you release your neck and upper back. Tuck your toes under, straighten your legs, and lift your knees off the floor.

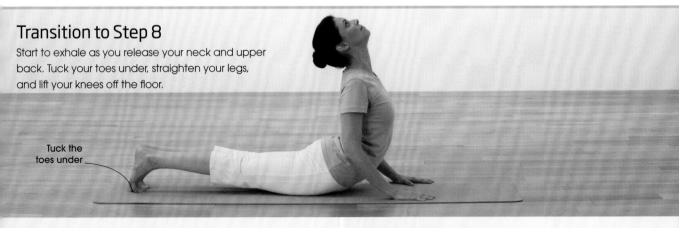

Tuck the toes under

8 Continue inhaling, lift your hips, straighten your arms, and push your body backward. Look at the floor.

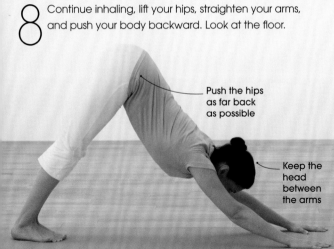

Push the hips as far back as possible

Keep the head between the arms

Transition to Step 9

Start to inhale as you step forward with your right leg, bringing your right foot between your hands and your right knee above your right ankle. Lower your left knee to the mat.

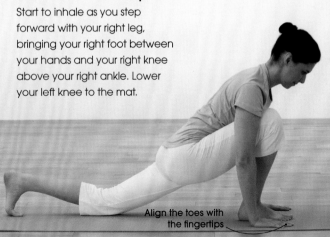

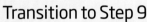

Align the toes with the fingertips

9 As you continue inhaling, stretch your left foot backward. Try to keep your hands flat on the mat. Look up and extend your neck and upper back. Keep your hips level. Keep your mouth closed.

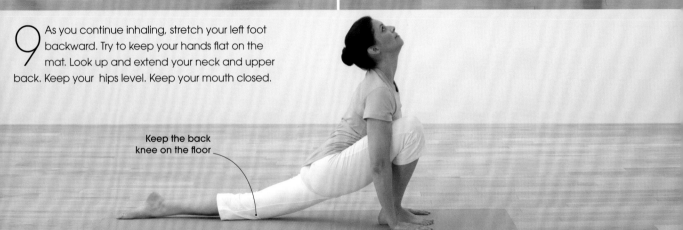

Keep the back knee on the floor

Sun Salutation
(continued)

Transition to Step 10

Start to exhale as you bring your left leg forward to meet the right, aligning your toes and fingertips and keeping your knees straight. Bend forward from the waist, but try not to bend your upper back. Look to the floor in front of you.

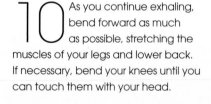

10 As you continue exhaling, bend forward as much as possible, stretching the muscles of your legs and lower back. If necessary, bend your knees until you can touch them with your head.

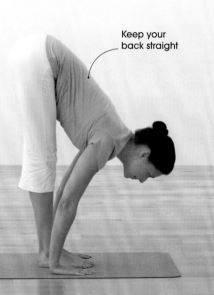

Keep your back straight

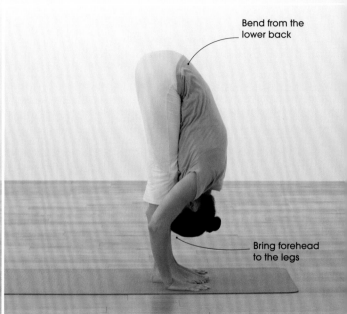

Bend from the lower back

Bring forehead to the legs

Transition (a) to Step 11

Start to inhale as you lift your spine forward from your waist, keeping your legs straight. Take your arms to your ears. Use the muscles of your back, shoulders, and neck to bring your spine, head, and arms into a horizontal line.

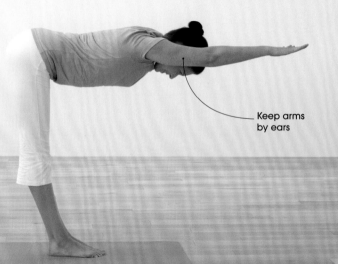

Keep arms by ears

Transition (b) to Step 11

Continuing to inhale, stretch your arms up to your ears, palms facing forward. As you lift your shoulders, avoid any tension in the neck.

11 Still continuing to inhale, take your weight onto your heels and look upward as you arch your arms, head, and chest backward. Stretch the muscles of your chest and abdomen.

12 Exhale as you lower your arms next to your body. Keep your spine upright and look straight ahead. Take a long inhalation, then continue with a second Sun Salutation, starting at Step 1. This time take your left knee to the mat in Step 4 and your right knee to the mat in Step 9.

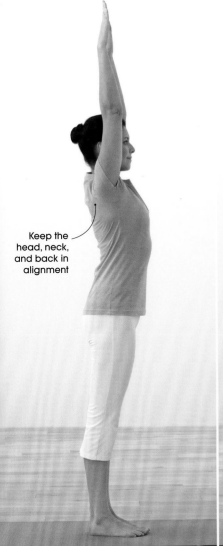

Keep the head, neck, and back in alignment

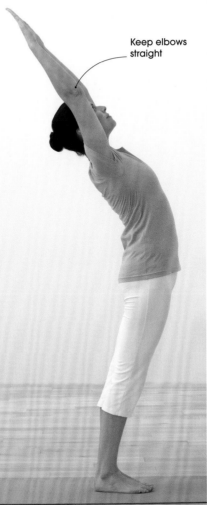

Keep elbows straight

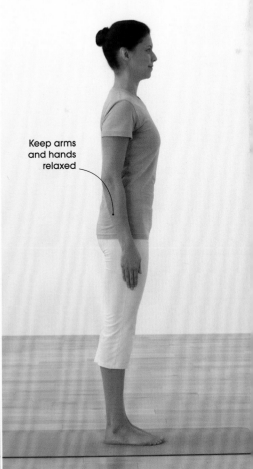

Keep arms and hands relaxed

Single Leg Lifts

All Levels

Single Leg Lifts improve the flexibility of the hamstring and calf muscles, which in turn helps prepare for the stretching of the back muscles in the various forward-bending asanas.

Single Leg Lift Beginner

1 Lie flat on your back with your legs together, arms next to your body, and palms face down.

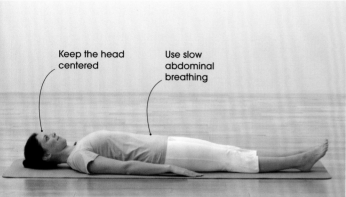

Keep the head centered

Use slow abdominal breathing

2 Inhale and raise your left leg, keeping your knee straight and your toes toward your head. Exhale and lower your leg back to the starting position. Repeat up to 5 times on each side, then continue with Head to Knee Raise or Deep Stretch Single Leg Lift.

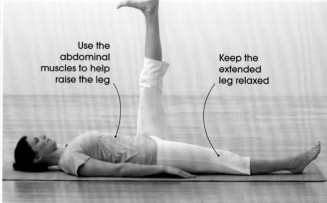

Use the abdominal muscles to help raise the leg

Keep the extended leg relaxed

Head to Knee Raise Beginner

1 Starting from Single Leg Lift Step 2 (see above), with an exhalation, bend your left leg and clasp your hands around your left knee, pushing your left thigh against your abdomen.

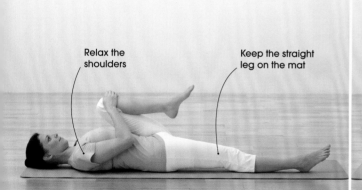

Relax the shoulders

Keep the straight leg on the mat

2 With an inhalation, lift your head and try to bring your forehead against your left knee. With an exhalation, lower your head, arms, and leg. Repeat on the opposite side. Practice up to 3 Head to Knee Raises on each side.

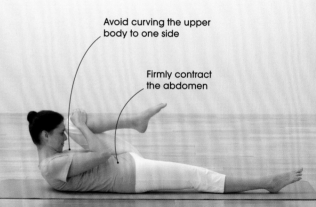

Avoid curving the upper body to one side

Firmly contract the abdomen

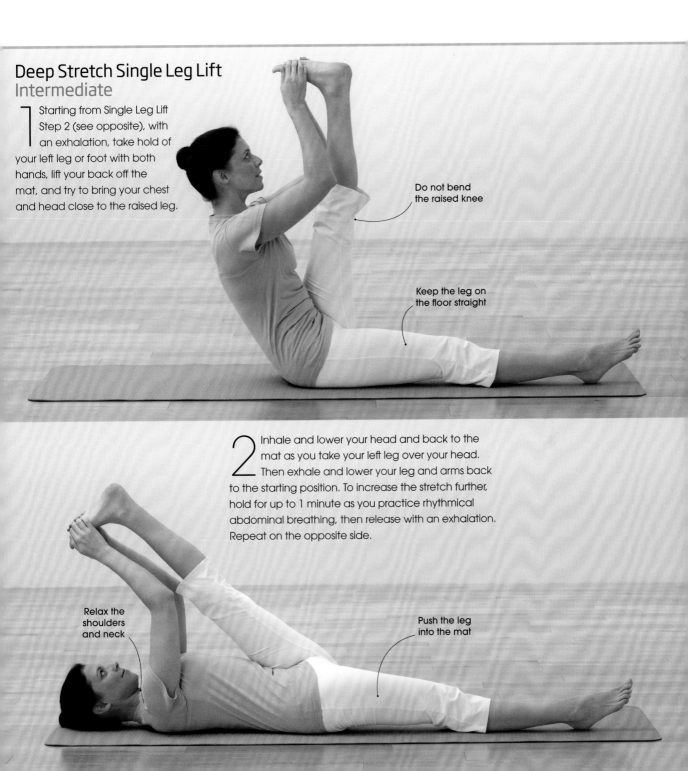

Deep Stretch Single Leg Lift
Intermediate

1 Starting from Single Leg Lift Step 2 (see opposite), with an exhalation, take hold of your left leg or foot with both hands, lift your back off the mat, and try to bring your chest and head close to the raised leg.

Do not bend the raised knee

Keep the leg on the floor straight

2 Inhale and lower your head and back to the mat as you take your left leg over your head. Then exhale and lower your leg and arms back to the starting position. To increase the stretch further, hold for up to 1 minute as you practice rhythmical abdominal breathing, then release with an exhalation. Repeat on the opposite side.

Relax the shoulders and neck

Push the leg into the mat

Double Leg Lifts
Intermediate and Advanced

These Double Leg Lifts provide abdominal strength, which is needed for many asanas, such as Headstand (see pp62–71). After doing Single, then Double Leg Lifts, relax in Corpse Pose (see p188).

Arms by Sides Intermediate

1 Lie flat on your back with your legs together, arms next to your body, and palms face down. Breathe slowly and rhythmically.

2 Tuck your arms under your body to prevent tension in your lower back, then inhale and lift both legs simultaneously to a 90-degree angle. With an exhalation, bring your legs back to the mat. Repeat 5–10 times. If you do not feel any tension in your lower back, practice with your arms by your sides, palms face down.

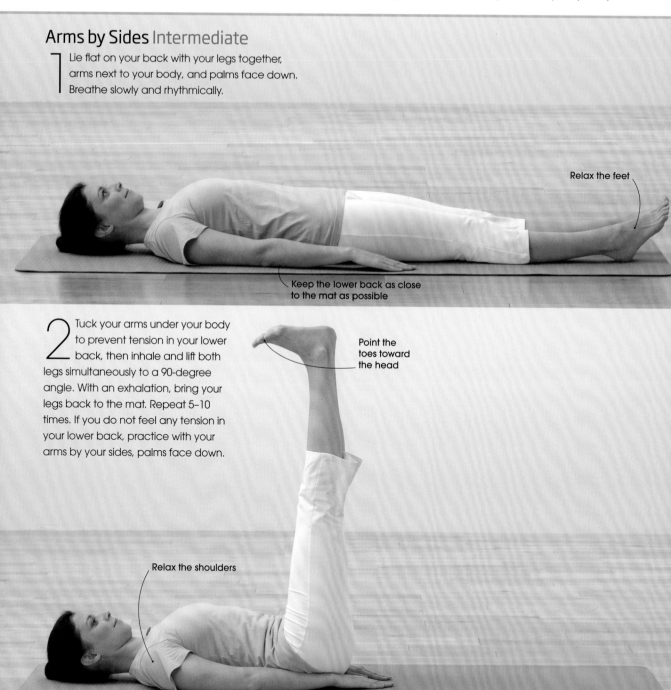

Relax the feet

Keep the lower back as close to the mat as possible

Point the toes toward the head

Relax the shoulders

Arms Overhead Advanced

1 Lie flat on your back, extend your arms on the floor behind you, and catch hold of your elbows. Breathe slowly and rhythmically.

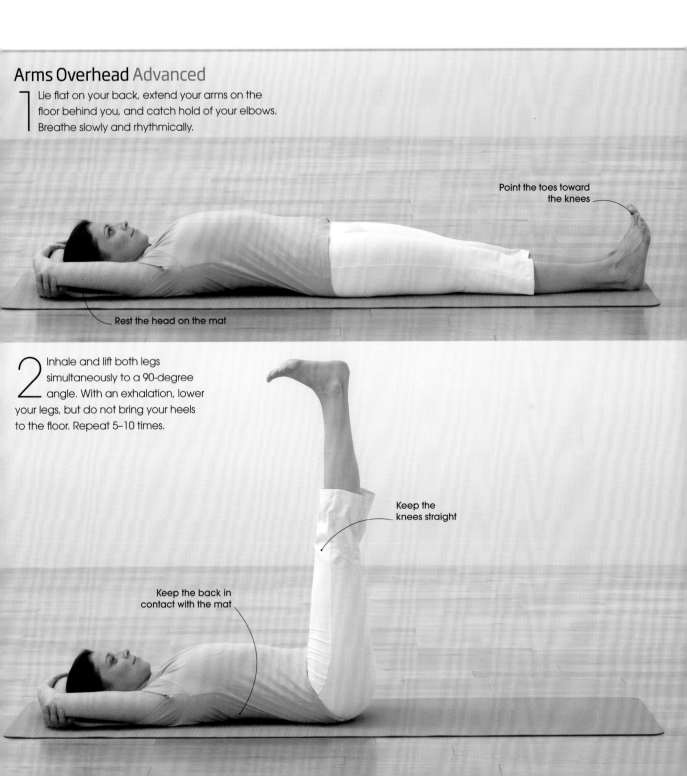

Point the toes toward the knees

Rest the head on the mat

2 Inhale and lift both legs simultaneously to a 90-degree angle. With an exhalation, lower your legs, but do not bring your heels to the floor. Repeat 5–10 times.

Keep the knees straight

Keep the back in contact with the mat

1 Headstand
Sirshasana

Headstand is a powerful pose for both body and mind. Balance in Headstand requires coordination of the impulses received in the brain from the inner ear, the skin of the arms and hands, the eyes, and various muscles and joints. Relax afterward in Child's Pose (see p191).

Benefits

PHYSICAL

- Creates a stronger heartbeat.
- Relieves varicose veins.
- Reduces pressure in the lower back.
- Helps to build muscle strength in the shoulder girdle.
- Improves the coordination of the body's voluntary and involuntary functions.

MENTAL

- Improves memory and concentration.
- Improves body-mind coordination.
- Enhances your intellectual capacities.

CAUTION Do not practice Headstand: If you suffer from high blood pressure; during menstruation; if you suffer from eye conditions such as detached retina or glaucoma; if you have any inflammation in the head area; if you suffer from neck pain due to an accident or other causes. If in doubt, consult your doctor.

Dolphin Preparatory Exercise for All Levels

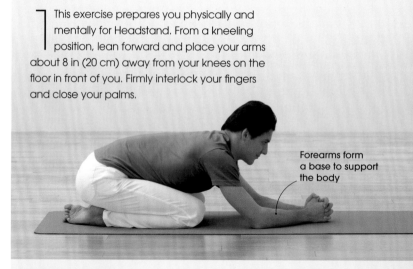

1 This exercise prepares you physically and mentally for Headstand. From a kneeling position, lean forward and place your arms about 8 in (20 cm) away from your knees on the floor in front of you. Firmly interlock your fingers and close your palms.

Forearms form a base to support the body

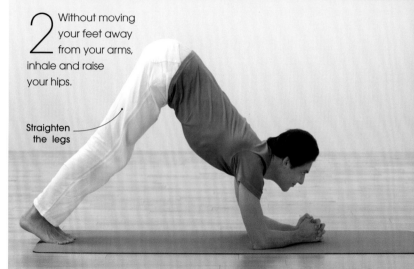

2 Without moving your feet away from your arms, inhale and raise your hips.

Straighten the legs

3 With an exhalation, rock your whole body forward and take your head and shoulders down toward the floor. Your hips will now be lower, too.

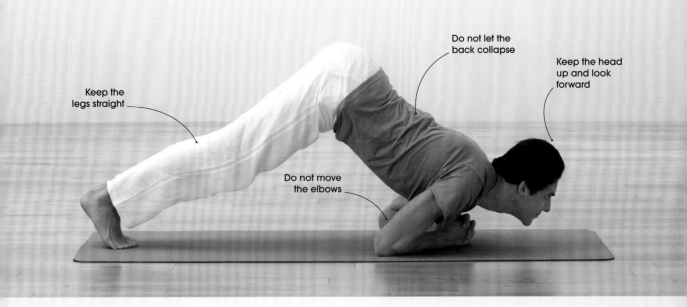

Do not let the back collapse

Keep the head up and look forward

Keep the legs straight

Do not move the elbows

4 Inhale and push your head and shoulders back up. Your hips will come back up, too. Repeat Steps 1–4 a total of 5–10 times, then bend your knees to the floor and relax in Child's Pose (see p191).

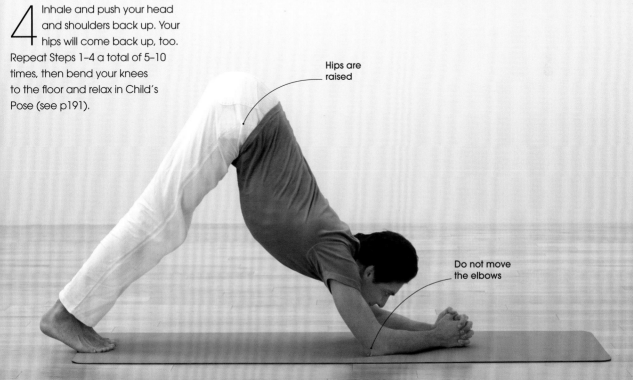

Hips are raised

Do not move the elbows

Headstand
Beginner

Think: "My arms are my legs." These are the instructions that Swami Vishnudevananda used to help students to focus on the tripod base formed by their elbows and hands in this pose.

STARTING POSITION Relax in Child's Pose (see p191) for a few moments before you practice Headstand.

1 Lean forward, clasping each hand around the opposite elbow and placing your arms about 8 in (20 cm) away from your knees on the floor in front of you.

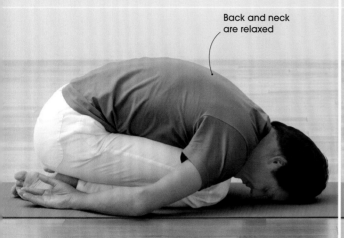

Back and neck are relaxed

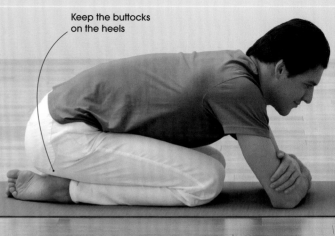

Keep the buttocks on the heels

2 Without changing the position of your elbows, interlock your fingers, keeping your palms open. Your hands and elbows provide the firm tripod base for your Headstand.

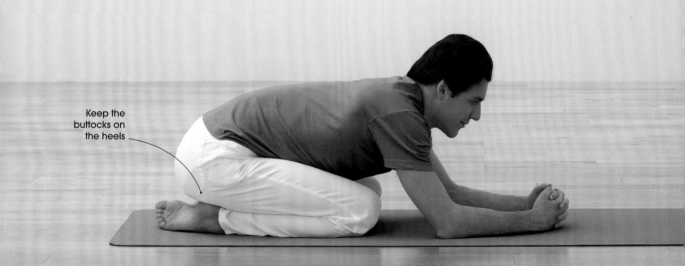

Keep the buttocks on the heels

3 Bend over and place the topmost part of your head on the floor, firmly pressing the tripod of elbows and hands against the mat.

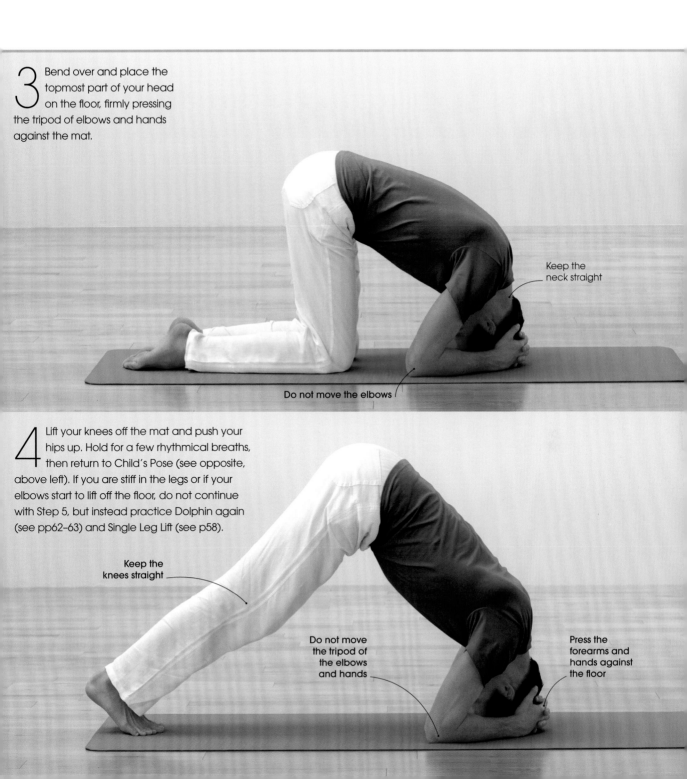

Keep the neck straight

Do not move the elbows

4 Lift your knees off the mat and push your hips up. Hold for a few rhythmical breaths, then return to Child's Pose (see opposite, above left). If you are stiff in the legs or if your elbows start to lift off the floor, do not continue with Step 5, but instead practice Dolphin again (see pp62–63) and Single Leg Lift (see p58).

Keep the knees straight

Do not move the tripod of the elbows and hands

Press the forearms and hands against the floor

Headstand
Intermediate and Advanced

You should not practice Headstand against a wall. The secret of success in this pose is to focus on the tripod base formed by your elbows and hands, and on the point of balance in your lower back.

Start with

Starting position p64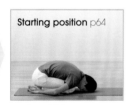

1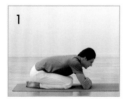

2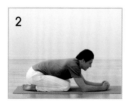

3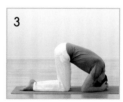

4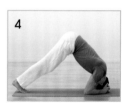

5 Starting from Headstand Step 4, and keeping your legs straight, walk your toes as close to your head as possible. Do not allow your back to collapse.

6 Breathing slowly and rhythmically, bend your legs and use your lower back muscles to pull your legs and pelvis up, until you are firmly balanced on your tripod base. Occasional contraction of your abdominal muscles will prevent you from falling over.

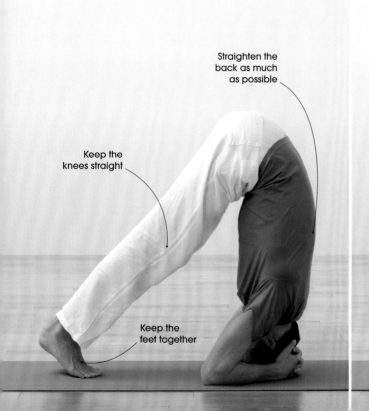

Straighten the back as much as possible

Keep the knees straight

Keep the feet together

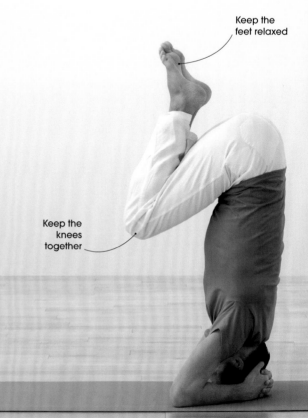

Keep the feet relaxed

Keep the knees together

"Sirshasana [Headstand] invigorates, energizes, and vivifies. It is a true blessing and a nectar. You will find real pleasure and exhilaration of spirit in this asana." Swami Sivananda

7 Continue to breathe rhythmically. Firmly press the tripod of elbows and hands against the floor. Focus on the point of balance in your lower back, then slowly start lifting your knees until your thighs are vertical and your feet are behind you.

Feel the point of balance in the lower back

Keep the legs together

Breathe rhythmically in the abdomen

Keep the shoulders away from the ears

8 To come into the full pose, extend your knees and take your legs straight up. Avoid any tension in your legs and feet. Hold for 1–5 minutes, then come down by following Steps 7–1, in that order. Relax in Child's Pose (see p191) for at least 6 deep breaths, then lie in Corpse Pose (see p188) for 1 minute.

COMMON FAULTS

Legs are not vertical

Lower back is curved

Neck is tense

Head is balancing on the forehead

Too much weight on the head

Fingers are too loose

Headstand
Variations

Each of these Headstand variations helps you to improve your balance, coordination, and powers of concentration. Move carefully until, in the end, your legs move as freely as if they were arms.

Start with

Starting position p64	1	2	3	4
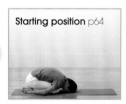	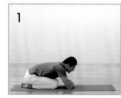	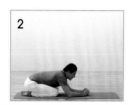	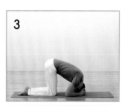	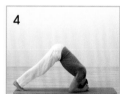

Legs to the Sides
Advanced

Starting from Headstand Step 8, with an exhalation, open your legs to the sides and let gravity pull them down toward the floor. Hold for up to 1 minute with deep, rhythmical breathing.

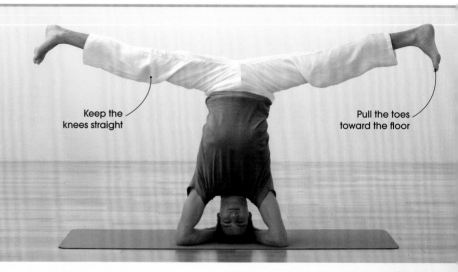

Keep the knees straight

Pull the toes toward the floor

Legs to Front and Back
Advanced

Starting from Headstand Step 8, with an exhalation, slowly take one leg forward and the other leg equally far back. Change legs. If your Headstand is well balanced, you can alternate your legs in a flowing rhythm, with deep, rhythmical breathing for up to 1 minute.

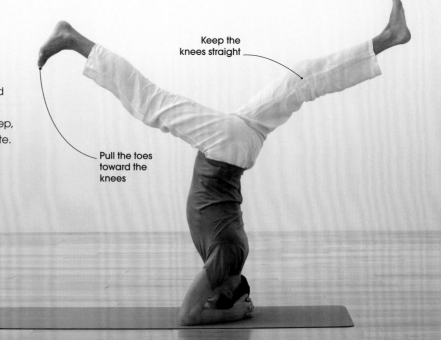

Keep the knees straight

Pull the toes toward the knees

After each variation, bring your legs back together into Headstand Step 8, then either practice another variation, or come down by doing Steps 7-1 in that order. Relax afterward in Child's Pose (see p191).

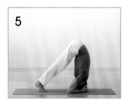
5

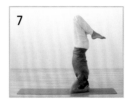
6

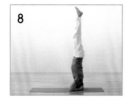
7

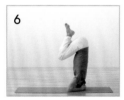
8

Knees Bent to the Sides Advanced

Starting from Headstand Step 8, with an exhalation, bend your knees to the sides and carefully bring the soles of your feet together. Hold for up to 1 minute with deep, rhythmical breathing.

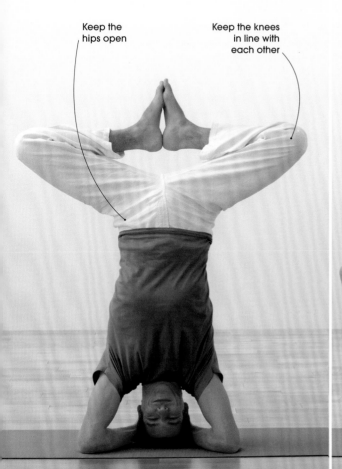

Keep the hips open

Keep the knees in line with each other

One Leg to the Ground
Advanced

Starting from Headstand Step 8, with an exhalation, lower your right leg toward the ground as far as you can. Inhale and raise the leg up again. Repeat on the opposite side, then continue, alternating sides, for up to 1 minute with deep, rhythmical breathing.

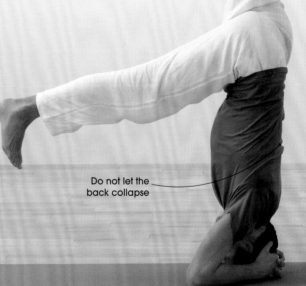

Keep the upper leg vertically aligned

Do not let the back collapse

Headstand
Variations (continued)

These advanced variations teach you to bend and twist in Headstand. Movements of the spine like these give your back an excellent workout—even while you are on your head.

Start with

Starting position p64	1	2	3	4

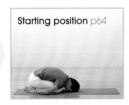 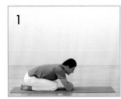 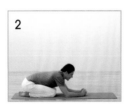 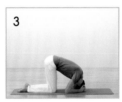 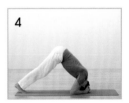

Both Legs to the Ground
Advanced

Starting from Headstand Step 8, with an exhalation and keeping your legs together, lower them in a controlled manner as far as possible toward the floor. With the next inhalation, bring the legs back up. Repeat the movement up to 5 times.

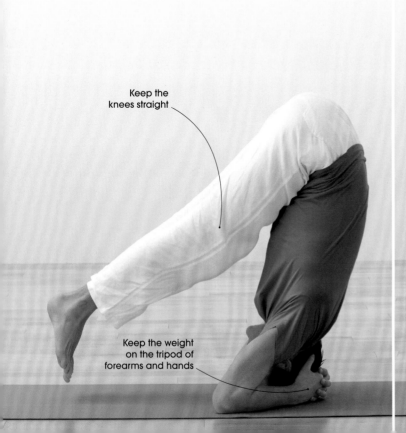

Keep the knees straight

Keep the weight on the tripod of forearms and hands

Lotus Headstand
Advanced

Starting from Headstand Step 8, with an exhalation, bring your legs into Lotus (see p114). Hold for up to 1 minute, breathing rhythmically, then uncross your legs, cross them the other way, and hold for up to 1 minute more.

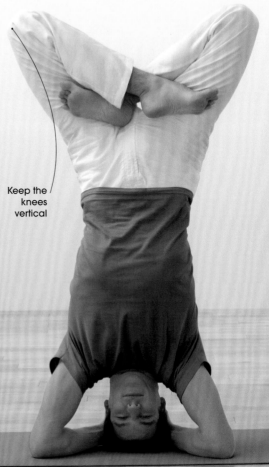

Keep the knees vertical

After each variation, bring your legs back together into Headstand Step 8, then either practice another variation, or come down by doing Steps 7-1 in that order. Relax afterward in Child's Pose (see p191).

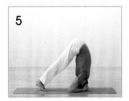 5

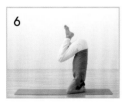 6

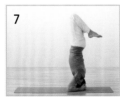 7

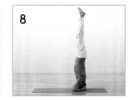 8

Twisted Lotus Headstand
Advanced

Starting from Lotus Headstand (see opposite), with an exhalation, twist your spine to one side. After a few breaths, slowly twist to the other side. Undo your legs, cross them the other way, and repeat.

Forward Bend Lotus Headstand
Advanced

Starting from Lotus Headstand (see opposite), with an exhalation, start bending forward from the hips. Hold for 3 breaths, with each exhalation trying to bend a little lower. Inhale and come back up into Lotus Headstand. Repeat twice more.

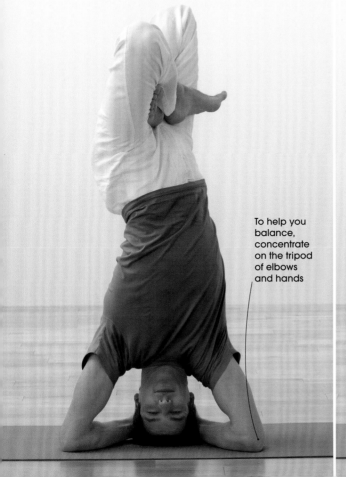

To help you balance, concentrate on the tripod of elbows and hands

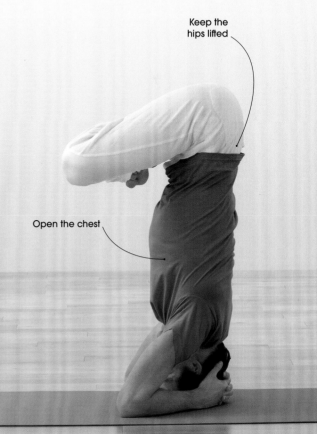

Keep the hips lifted

Open the chest

Scorpion
Advanced

Once you feel secure in Headstand and can hold it for at least 2 minutes, you can attempt Scorpion. Get used to arching your body backward. You will soon be balancing in Scorpion.

Start with

Starting position p64

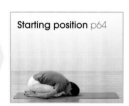

1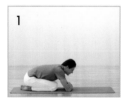

2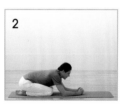

3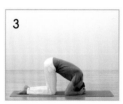

4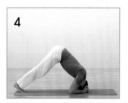

9 Starting from Headstand Step 8, press down on the tripod base formed by your elbows and hands. With an exhalation, bend your body backward as you push your hips forward.

10 Staying firm in your forearms and shoulders, and breathing deeply and rhythmically, separate your hands to about shoulder-width apart. Place your palms flat on the floor either side of your head.

11 To come into the full pose, with an inhalation, lift your head and find your balance on your forearms. Hold the pose for up to 30 seconds.

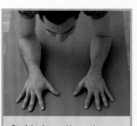

Stable base Keep the forearms almost parallel to each other and the fingers spread as widely as possible.

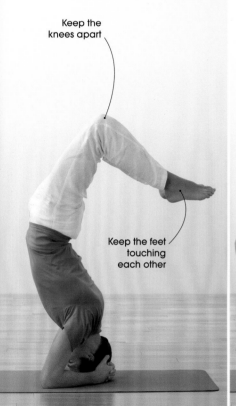

Keep the knees apart

Keep the feet touching each other

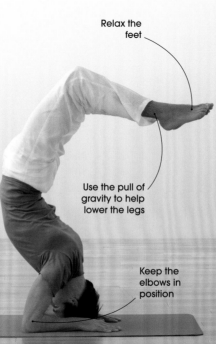

Relax the feet

Use the pull of gravity to help lower the legs

Keep the elbows in position

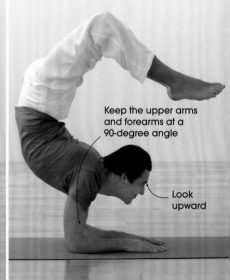

Keep the upper arms and forearms at a 90-degree angle

Look upward

After practicing Scorpion or its variations, return to Headstand Step 8, then either practice another variation, or come down by doing Steps 7–1 in that order. Relax afterward in Child's Pose (see p191).

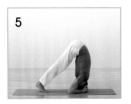

5

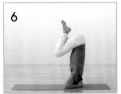

6

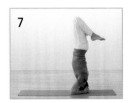

7

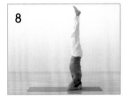

8

Straight Legs Variation

Starting from Scorpion Step 11 (see opposite), with an inhalation, straighten your legs. The more you move your legs forward over your head, the more you have to direct your head and eyes upward. Hold for up to 30 seconds.

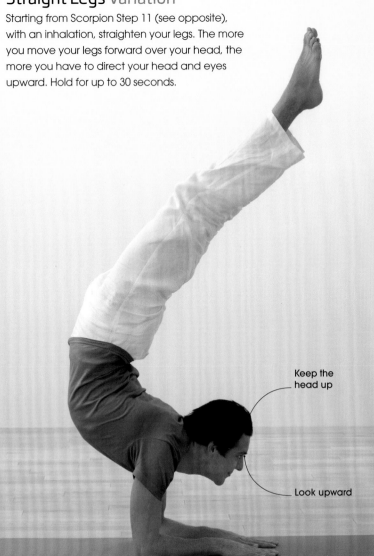

Keep the head up

Look upward

Feet to Head Variation

Starting from Scorpion Step 11 (see opposite), with a series of strong exhalations, bend your spine and legs until your feet touch your head. Keep your knees apart to reduce the pressure on your lower back. Hold for up to 30 seconds.

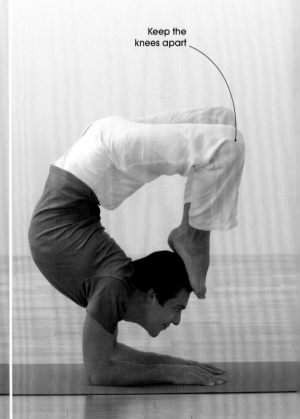

Keep the knees apart

Handstand
Advanced

Practice Handstand against a wall until you are confident enough to balance on your hands and arms. Handstand offers all the benefits of Headstand, without putting weight on your head.

1 Step one foot in front of the other, then bend forward and place both hands firmly on the mat, about shoulder-width apart. Keep your back straight and make sure that you do not allow your head to drop.

2 On an exhalation, swing your left leg up, followed by your right leg. This involves a pulling motion on your upper leg as you swing it up, and a pushing motion on your lower leg as you jump into position. Stay firm in your arms and hands.

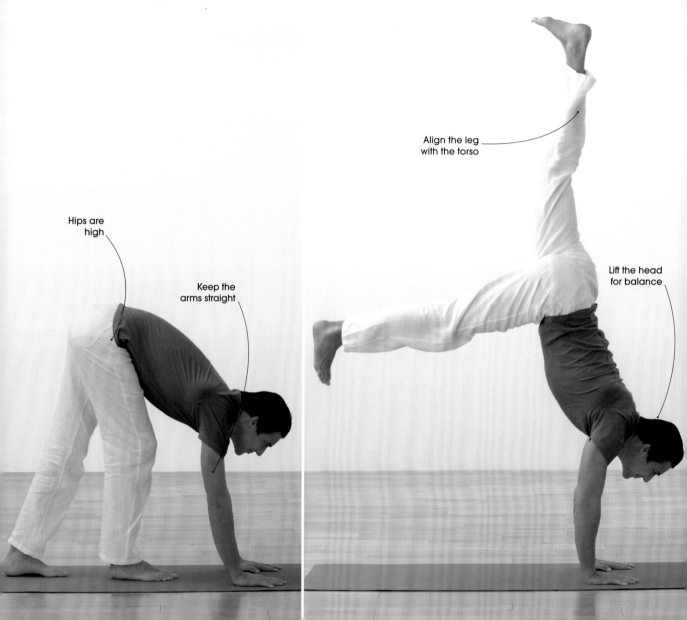

Align the leg with the torso

Hips are high

Keep the arms straight

Lift the head for balance

3 Keep both legs together as you balance in the full pose. Hold the pose for a few breaths, then come down by bringing one leg at a time to the floor. Relax in Child's Pose (see p191).

Scorpion Handstand
Variation

Starting from Handstand Step 3 (see left), bend your spine and legs to bring your feet toward your head. If you are very flexible, you should be able to touch your head with your feet. Come out of the pose by raising your feet back into Handstand, then bringing one leg at a time down to the floor. Relax in Child's Pose (see p191).

Keep the knees straight

Bend the back as little as possible

Separate the legs

Relax the legs to allow gravity to pull them down

Lift the head as high as possible

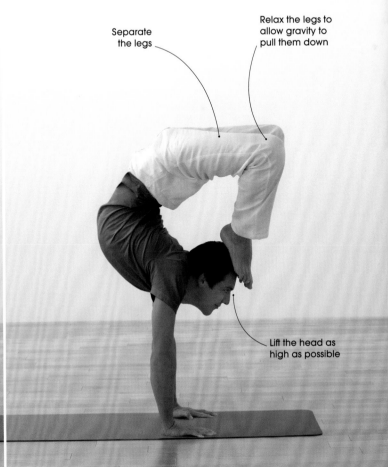

2 Shoulderstand
Sarvangasana

The pressure of the chin against the chest and the inversion of the body in Shoulderstand create the energy flow of Hatha yoga—the union in the solar plexus of the ascending sun energy "Ha" with the descending moon energy, or "Tha." Always practice Fish (see pp92–93) as the counterpose, then relax in Corpse Pose (see p188).

Benefits

PHYSICAL

- Tones and revitalizes the thyroid and parathyroid glands. This improves and balances the metabolism of literally every cell in the body.
- Improves the blood supply to the roots of the spinal nerves.
- Stretches away any stress held in the shoulder and neck area.
- Relieves the pain of varicose veins.

MENTAL

- Stimulates cheerfulness and helps to cure depression.
- Helps to relieve mental sluggishness and promotes clear thinking.

CAUTION If you suffer from high blood pressure, do not hold the pose for more than 30 seconds. If you have a slipped disc or other painful neck condition, practice only as far as Step 3.

Shoulderstand Beginner

1 Lie flat on your back with your legs together, arms next to your body, and palms touching the mat. Breathe rhythmically in your abdomen.

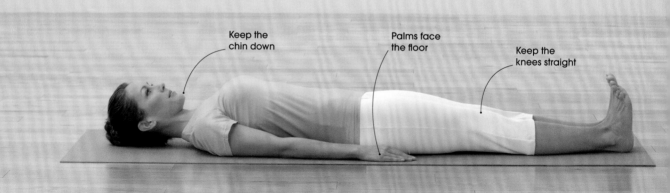

Keep the chin down

Palms face the floor

Keep the knees straight

2 Keeping your back, head, and neck on the mat, inhale and, with your legs straight, lift them to a 90-degree angle.

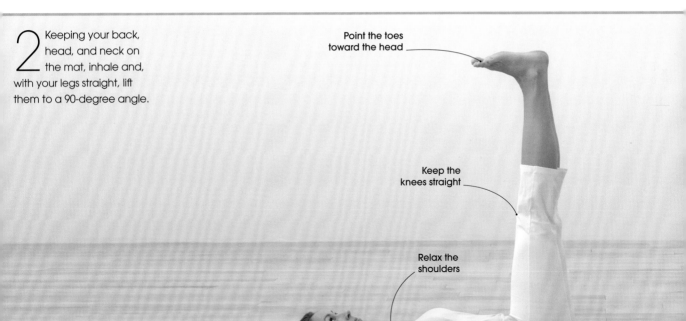

Point the toes toward the head

Keep the knees straight

Relax the shoulders

Keep the head centered

3 On another inhalation, gently lift your legs and hips until you can place your hands flat against your lower back. Hold for a few rhythmical breaths, then come down by following the instructions on p79. Relax for at least 8 breaths in Corpse Pose (see p188).

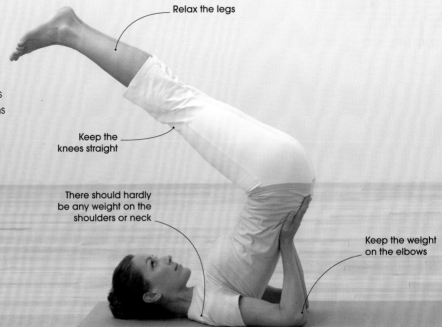

Relax the legs

Keep the knees straight

There should hardly be any weight on the shoulders or neck

Keep the weight on the elbows

Shoulderstand
Intermediate and Advanced

As you progress in Shoulderstand, the more you will be able to align the legs, hips, and back, making it easier to hold the pose, since the back muscles will not need to work so hard against gravity.

Start with

1 p76

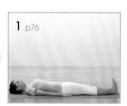

2

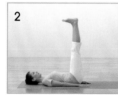

3

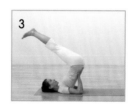

4 To come into the final pose, start from Shoulderstand Step 3. Continue lifting your body until your legs are in a straight line, and bring your chin as close to your chest as possible. Hold for up to 3 minutes.

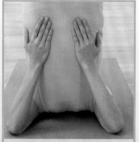

Hand position Take your hands as close as possible to your shoulder blades, with your arms as parallel to each other as possible.

Make sure the feet are relaxed

Breathe rhythmically in the abdomen

Maintain a constant pressure of the hands and arms against the upper back

COMMON FAULTS

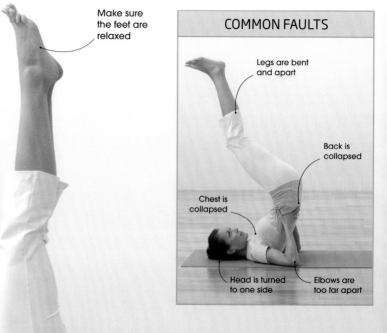

Legs are bent and apart

Back is collapsed

Chest is collapsed

Head is turned to one side

Elbows are too far apart

TO COME DOWN, slowly place both arms flat on the floor, palms face down, and bend your hips, bringing both legs slightly behind you, toward the floor. Using your arms as a brake, slowly roll down, vertebra by vertebra. Once your back is flat on the mat, use your abdominal muscles to lower your legs. Relax for at least 8 breaths in Corpse Pose (see p188).

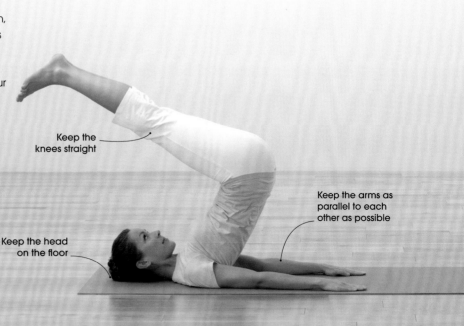

Keep the knees straight

Keep the arms as parallel to each other as possible

Keep the head on the floor

Arms on Floor
Advanced Variation

Starting from Shoulderstand Step 4, slowly place both arms flat on the floor, palms face down. Keep your body upright. Hold for up to 1 minute, then come down by following the instructions above. Relax for at least 8 breaths in Corpse Pose (see p188).

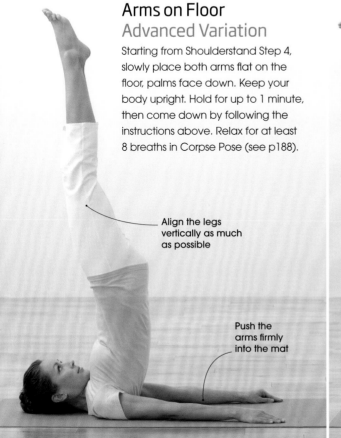

Align the legs vertically as much as possible

Push the arms firmly into the mat

Hands on Thighs
Advanced Variation

Starting from Shoulderstand Step 4, slowly lift one arm at a time and take it onto the front of your thigh. Keep your balance on your shoulders, neck, and head. Hold for up to 1 minute, then come down by following the instructions above. Relax for at least 8 breaths in Corpse Pose (see p188).

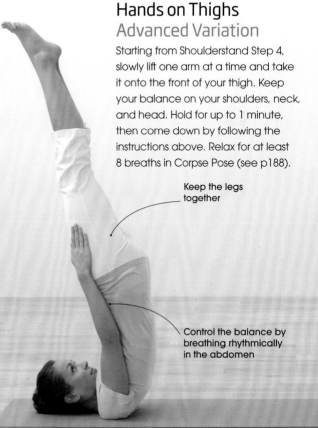

Keep the legs together

Control the balance by breathing rhythmically in the abdomen

3 Plough
Halasana

Plough is a natural continuation of the forward-bending movement you did in Shoulderstand (see pp76–79). The shape you make, with your feet and hands on the floor, resembles a plough. This asana helps to keep the whole spine youthful. Relax afterward in Corpse Pose (see p188) for at least 8 breaths.

Benefits

PHYSICAL

- Stretches the back of the body completely, which mobilizes the entire spine.
- Loosens tight hamstrings.
- Stretches the deep and superficial muscles of the back.
- Increases the blood supply to the nerves of the spine.
- Releases tension in the shoulder and neck muscles.

- Helps improve the flexibility of the shoulder joint.
- Improves digestion and helps to overcome constipation by placing pressure on the abdominal area.

MENTAL

- By teaching you how to breathe and relax while there is pressure on the front of your body, Plough helps you cope better with any claustrophobia, stress, or sense of being overwhelmed by a lack of space in your daily life.

CAUTION If you are suffering from an acute slipped disc, you should consult your doctor or physiotherapist before starting this exercise.

Plough Beginner

1 Lie flat on your back with your legs together, arms next to your body, and palms face down on the mat.

Keep the legs together

2 With an inhalation, slowly start lifting both your legs to a 90-degree angle. Keep your arms, head, and shoulders on the floor.

Point the toes toward the head

Keep the knees straight

3 With another inhalation, lift your legs and hips until you can place your hands against your lower back.

Keep the toes pointed toward the head

Keep the weight on the elbows

4 With an exhalation, slowly lower your legs behind your head, taking your feet to the floor. If your feet do not reach the floor, hold this pose for 5 breaths, then roll out as described on p83 and relax on your back. Once your feet do reach the floor, continue with Step 5 (see p82).

Make sure the knees are straight

Keep the back supported with the hands

Keep the toes pointing toward the head

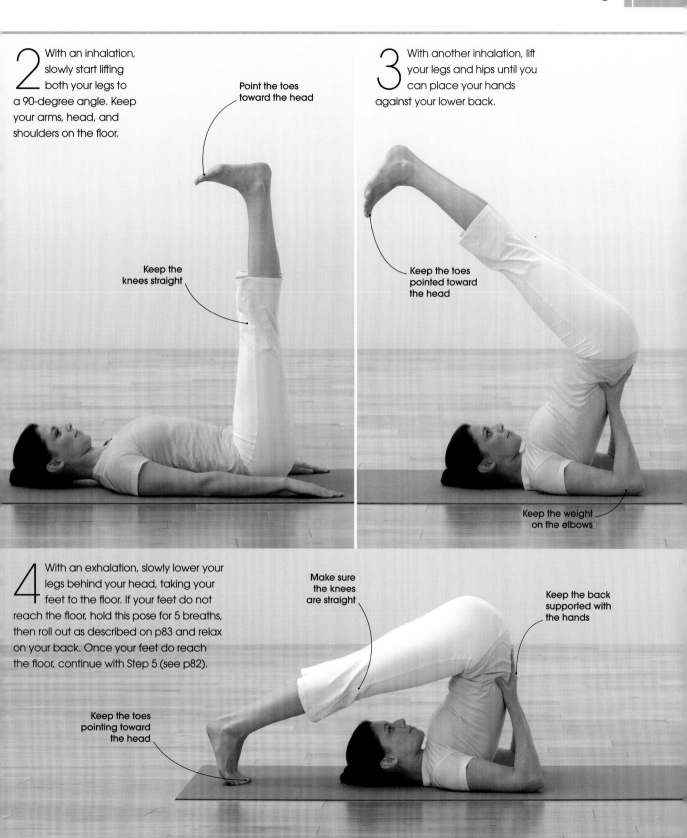

Plough
Intermediate and Advanced

At the intermediate level of Plough you hyperextend your arms as you place them on the floor. This increases your flexibility, not only in your hips and back, but also in your shoulder girdle.

Start with

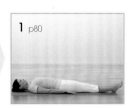

1 p80

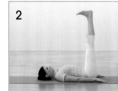

2

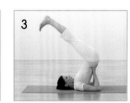

3

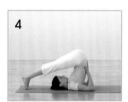

4

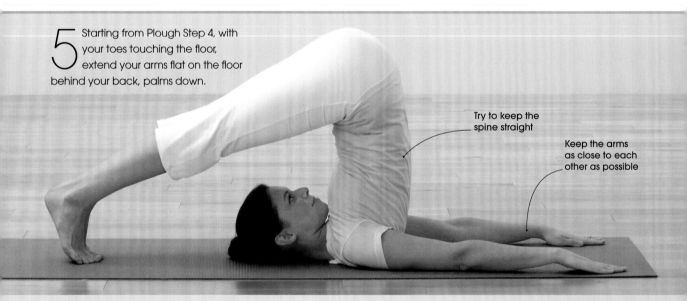

5 Starting from Plough Step 4, with your toes touching the floor, extend your arms flat on the floor behind your back, palms down.

Try to keep the spine straight

Keep the arms as close to each other as possible

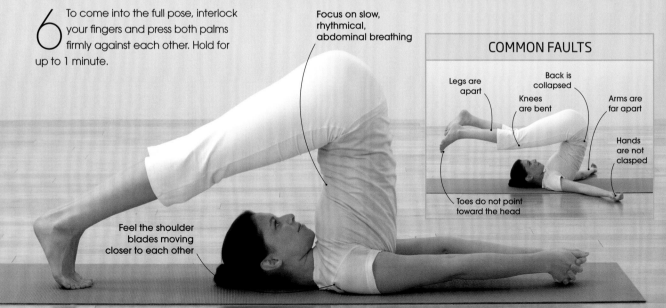

6 To come into the full pose, interlock your fingers and press both palms firmly against each other. Hold for up to 1 minute.

Focus on slow, rhythmical, abdominal breathing

Feel the shoulder blades moving closer to each other

COMMON FAULTS

Legs are apart

Back is collapsed

Knees are bent

Arms are far apart

Hands are not clasped

Toes do not point toward the head

*"Never behold life physically.
Understand it psychically,
and realize it spiritually."* Swami Sivananda

TO COME OUT of the pose, release your hands, place your arms flat on the floor and raise your legs until they are parallel to the floor. With an exhalation, slowly roll down to the floor, vertebra by vertebra. Relax for at least 8 breaths in Corpse Pose (see p188).

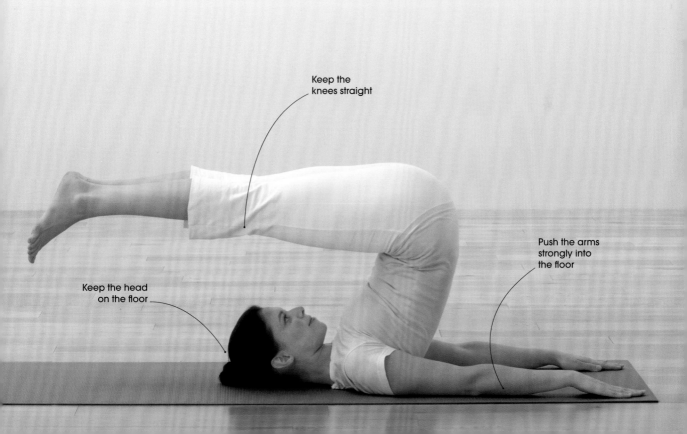

Keep the
knees straight

Push the arms
strongly into
the floor

Keep the head
on the floor

Plough
Variations

As well as working the hips and giving the upper back a deep stretch, these Plough variations give the solar plexus a powerful massage—as long as you keep up your rhythmical breathing.

Start with

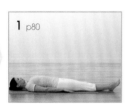

1 p80

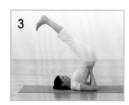

2

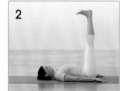

3

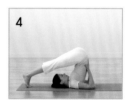

4

Feet Apart Beginner

Starting from Plough Step 4, keep your knees straight as you take your legs as far apart as possible. Extend your hands flat on the floor behind you, palms face down. Hold for up to 1 minute, then raise your legs until they are parallel to the floor. Continue coming out of the pose and relaxing as described on p83.

Keep the back as straight as possible

Push the heels toward the floor

Arm Wrap Intermediate

Starting from Feet Apart (see above), lower your knees next to your ears. Bring your arms over your knees and take your hands to your ears. Hold for up to 1 minute, breathing slowly, then come out of the pose and relax as described on p83.

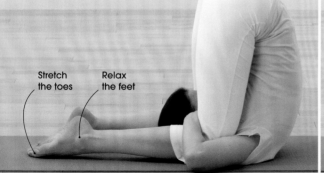

Stretch the toes

Relax the feet

Hands to Feet Intermediate

Starting from Plough Step 4, take your arms next to your ears and try to touch your toes. Hold for up to 1 minute, breathing slowly, then come out of the pose and relax as described on p83.

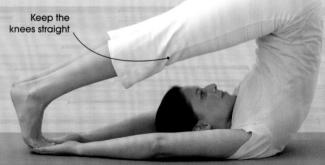

Keep the knees straight

"The self-effort of today becomes the destiny of tomorrow. Self-effort and destiny are one and the same." Swami Sivananda

Knees Behind Head Advanced

Starting from Plough Step 4, walk your feet as far away from your head as possible. Then bend your knees and slowly lower them to the mat behind your head. Hold for up to 30 seconds, then raise your legs until they are parallel to the floor. Continue coming out of the pose and relaxing as described on p83.

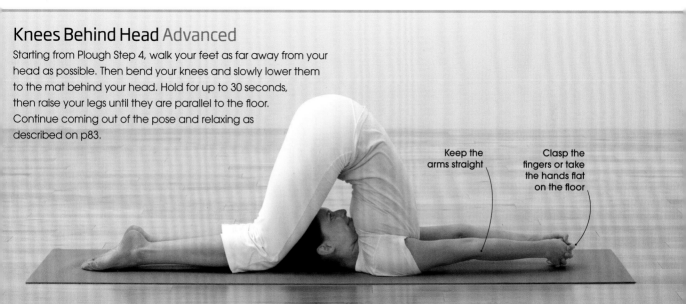

Keep the arms straight

Clasp the fingers or take the hands flat on the floor

Knees to Shoulder Advanced

1 Starting from Plough Step 4, support your back firmly with both hands. Walk both legs to the left side.

Keep the shoulders and elbows on the floor

2 Take both knees to the floor next to your left ear. Hold for up to 30 seconds, breathing slowly, then straighten your legs and bring your feet back to the center. Repeat on the other side, then come out of the pose and relax as described on p83.

Relax the toes and feet

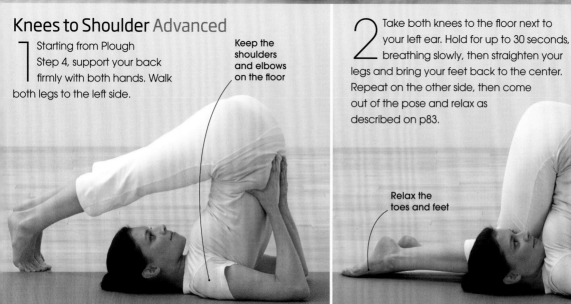

Bridge
All Levels

Bridge improves both the flexibility and strength of your spine in one extremely elegant pose. Steps 2–4 also provide an excellent training program for progressively strengthening your wrists.

Beginner

1 Lie on your back, with your feet and legs about 20 in (50 cm) apart, your knees bent, and your feet flat on the floor. Place your arms by your sides, palms face down.

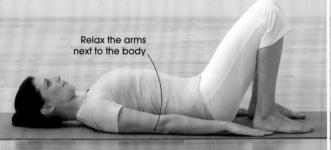

Relax the arms next to the body

2 Firmly catch hold of your ankles, inhale, and push your hips up.

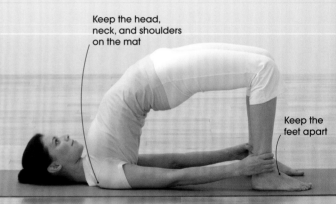

Keep the head, neck, and shoulders on the mat

Keep the feet apart

3 Release your hands and place them flat on your back, as close to your shoulder blades as possible. Point your fingers toward your lower back and place your thumbs on your sides. Breathe slowly and deeply. Either continue with Step 4 or come out by releasing your hands and lowering your hips. Then relax in Corpse Pose (see p188).

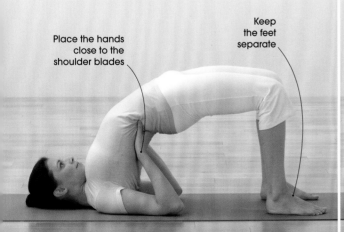

Place the hands close to the shoulder blades

Keep the feet separate

Intermediate

4 Come into the full pose by walking your feet farther away. Hold for up to 30 seconds, breathing deeply. Come out of the pose by walking your feet back toward your body, then release your hands and lower your hips. Relax in Corpse Pose (see p188).

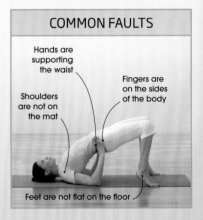

COMMON FAULTS

Hands are supporting the waist

Fingers are on the sides of the body

Shoulders are not on the mat

Feet are not flat on the floor

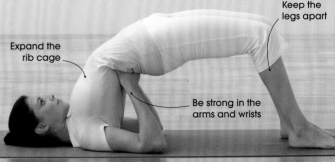

Expand the rib cage

Keep the legs apart

Be strong in the arms and wrists

Start with

1 p76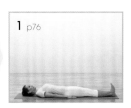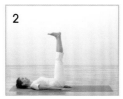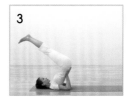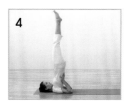

Shoulderstand to Bridge
Intermediate Variation

5 Once you have mastered Bridge, try coming into the pose from Shoulderstand Step 4. In this intermediate starting position, push your hands firmly against your back, bend both knees, and keep one leg over your head as you lower the other leg. Then lower the second leg to the floor, keeping your hips up. After a few breaths in Bridge, walk your feet closer to your body and, on an inhalation, lift one leg and then the other back up into Shoulderstand. Come out of the pose as described on p79 and relax.

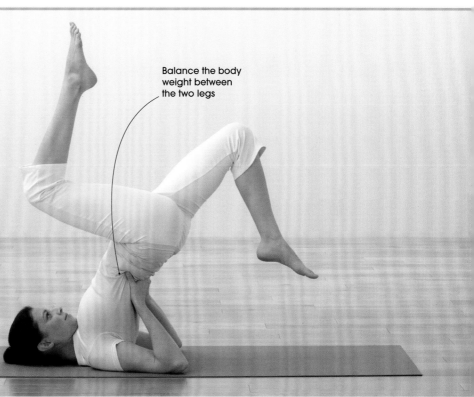

Balance the body weight between the two legs

Shoulderstand to Bridge
Advanced Variation

5 In this advanced starting position, begin with Shoulderstand Step 4, then bend your knees and lower both feet to the floor simultaneously. After a few breaths in Bridge, walk your feet closer to your body and, on an inhalation, lift one leg and then the other back up into Shoulderstand. Come out of the pose as described on p79 and relax.

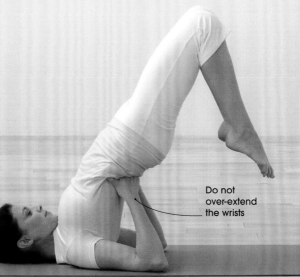

Do not over-extend the wrists

Bridge
Variations

After you have practiced these advanced Bridge variations, you should go back into Shoulderstand (see pp76–79) for up to 30 seconds before relaxing in Corpse Pose (see p188).

Start with

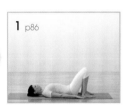
1 p86

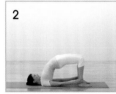
2

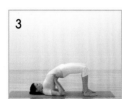
3

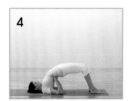
4

Single Leg Lift Advanced

Starting from Bridge Step 4, lift your left leg straight up as you inhale. After a few deep breaths, lower the leg with an exhalation, then repeat with your right leg. Come out of the pose by releasing your hands and lowering your hips, then relax in Corpse Pose (see p188).

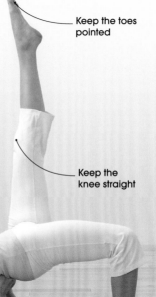

Keep the toes pointed

Keep the knee straight

Keep the neck and the shoulders on the mat

Legs Straight Advanced

Starting from Bridge Step 4, bring your legs and feet together, then walk your feet away until your legs are completely straight. Hold for up to 30 seconds, breathing deeply. Come out of the pose by walking your feet closer to your body, releasing your hands, and lowering your hips. Relax in Corpse Pose (see p188).

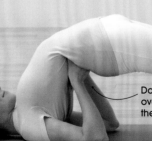

Do not over-extend the wrists

Start with

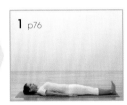 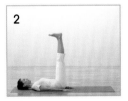 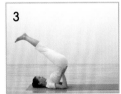 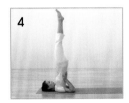

1 p76   2   3   4

Half Lotus Bridge Advanced

5 Starting from Shoulderstand Step 4, bend your left leg and use your right hand to pull your left foot closer to your hip.

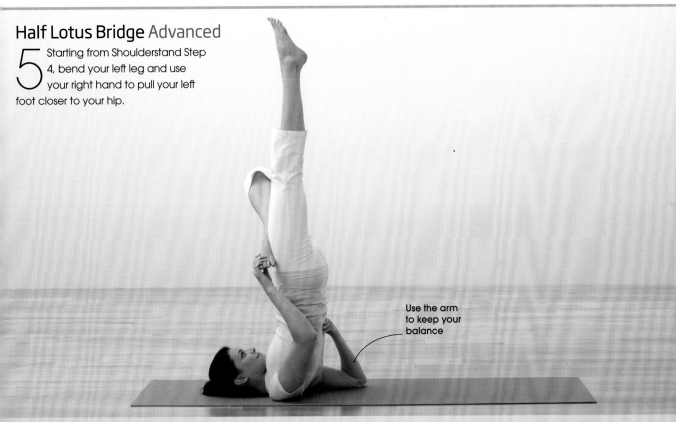

Use the arm to keep your balance

6 Support your back with both hands and slowly bring your right foot down to the floor. Hold for up to 30 seconds, then try to kick back up into Shoulderstand. If you cannot do this, lower your left foot to the floor, release your hands, lower your hips, then inhale and return to Shoulderstand Step 4. Repeat on the opposite side. If you can kick back up into Shoulderstand, come out of the pose as described on p79. Otherwise release your hands and lower your hips. Relax in Corpse Pose (see p188).

Bring the knee into a horizontal position

Walk the foot away from the body

Shoulderstand Cycle
Intermediate

The Shoulderstand Cycle is an excellent exercise for strengthening the muscles of the arms, the back, the abdomen, and the wrists. It also helps you to improve your alignment in Shoulderstand.

Start with

1 p80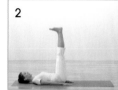

2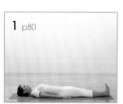

3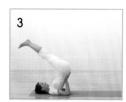

4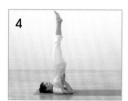

5 Starting with Shoulderstand Step 4, position your arms and hands firmly.

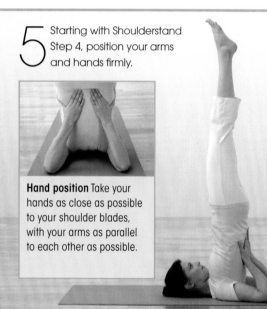

Hand position Take your hands as close as possible to your shoulder blades, with your arms as parallel to each other as possible.

6 On an exhalation, come into Single Leg Plough by lowering your left leg over your head until your toes reach the floor. Inhale and bring your leg back. Repeat, lowering your right leg.

Keep the upper leg straight and vertical

7 On an exhalation, transition into Plough by lowering both legs over your head until your toes reach the floor.

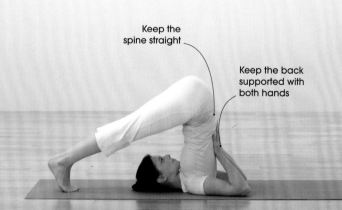

Keep the spine straight

Keep the back supported with both hands

8 Come back into Shoulderstand by lifting both legs simultaneously on an inhalation. If you find this difficult, you may move your hips forward slightly, then lift your legs. This lessens the impact of the weight of your legs on your back muscles.

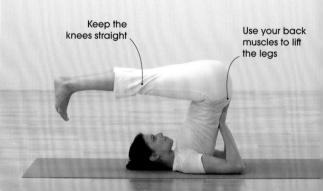

Keep the knees straight

Use your back muscles to lift the legs

"Health is Wealth.
Peace of Mind is Happiness.
Yoga shows the Way." Swami Vishnudevananda

9 Once you are in Shoulderstand, breathe deeply, bring your elbows closer, and take your hands as close to your shoulder blades as possible.

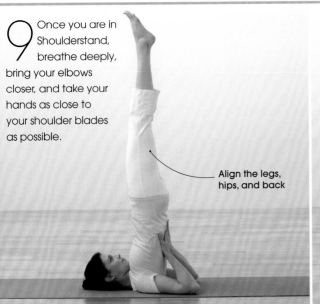

Align the legs, hips, and back

10 Transition into Bridge by bending both knees and keeping one leg over your head as you lower the other leg to the floor.

Balance the weight between both legs

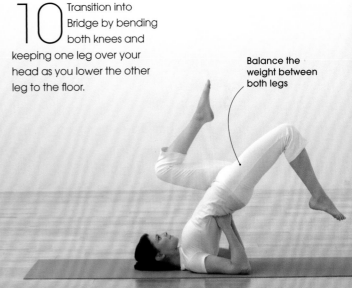

11 In Bridge, continue supporting your back. With your legs still apart, walk your feet farther away. Breathe rhythmically.

Keep the arms and wrists firm

Expand the rib cage

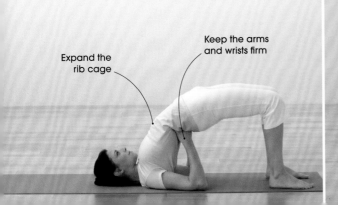

12 Come back into Shoulderstand by walking your feet closer to your body. On an inhalation, lift one leg straight up, push firmly on the opposite leg, and lift your body back up into Shoulderstand. Breathe slowly and rhythmically. Repeat the cycle 1–2 times more, then come out of the pose as described on p79 and relax.

4 Fish
Matsyasana

Fish bends your spine in the opposite direction to Shoulderstand (see pp76-79) and is the counterpose to the Shoulderstand Cycle. Spend at least half as much time doing Fish as you do Shoulderstand. After practicing Fish, you will find that you experience a deeper relaxation in Corpse Pose (see p188).

Benefits

PHYSICAL

• Relieves stiffness in the neck and shoulders.

• Corrects any tendency to round the shoulders.

• Strengthens the arm muscles.

• Expands the rib cage.

• Helps to tone the nerves of the neck and back area.

• Together with Shoulderstand, helps to improve the functioning of the thyroid and parathyroid glands.

• Improves the capacity of the lungs.

• Decongests the lungs.

• Relieves asthma.

MENTAL

• The wide opening of the rib cage reduces the pressure on the abdomen and recharges the solar plexus. This helps to overcome depression.

CAUTION If the hyper-extension of the neck causes any discomfort or dizziness, do not practice the posture or practice it for only a few breaths.

Fish Beginner and Intermediate

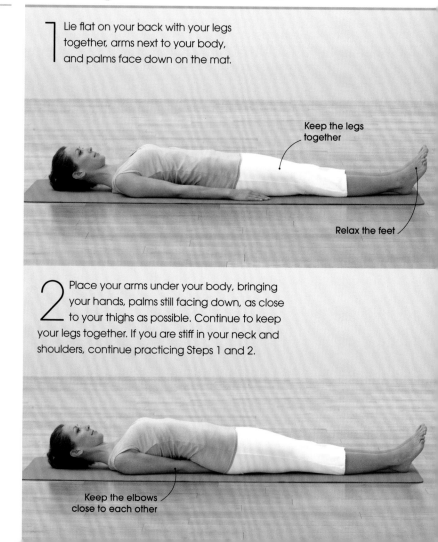

1 Lie flat on your back with your legs together, arms next to your body, and palms face down on the mat.

Keep the legs together

Relax the feet

2 Place your arms under your body, bringing your hands, palms still facing down, as close to your thighs as possible. Continue to keep your legs together. If you are stiff in your neck and shoulders, continue practicing Steps 1 and 2.

Keep the elbows close to each other

3 On an inhalation, bend your elbows and lift your chest as high as you can. Slowly extend your neck and head backward. Hold for a couple of deep breaths.

Relax the neck

While in the pose, breathe with a full yogic breath (see p181)

Keep the weight on the elbows

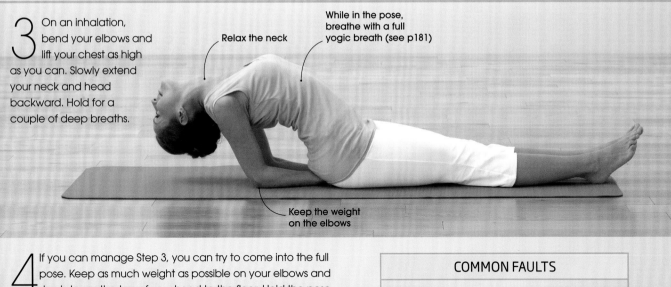

4 If you can manage Step 3, you can try to come into the full pose. Keep as much weight as possible on your elbows and slowly lower the top of your head to the floor. Hold the pose for half the time that you spent in Shoulderstand (see pp76–79). Come out of the pose by following Steps 3, 2, and 1 in that order.

COMMON FAULTS

Too much weight on the head

Chest is too low

Feet are apart

Elbows are too far apart

Hands are too high

Put as little weight on the head as possible

Keep the weight on the elbows

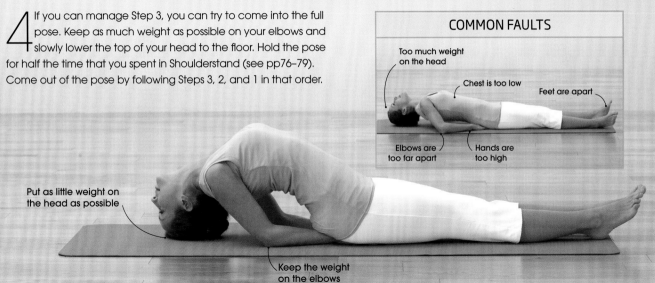

NECK STRETCH After doing Fish, practice this pose to release any tension in your neck. With your fingers interlocked behind your head and your forearms close to your ears, inhale and lift your head, pushing your chin into your chest. On an exhalation, slowly lower your head back to the mat. Repeat 2 times. Relax for 1–2 minutes in Corpse Pose (see p188).

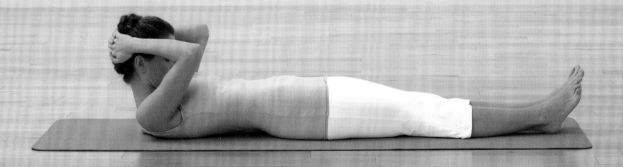

Fish
Variations

Cross-Legged Fish adds a deep thigh stretch, while Lotus Fish gives you a stable base, allowing you to intensify the backward bend. End each pose with the Neck Stretch (see p93).

Cross-Legged Fish Intermediate

1 Lie on your back, cross your legs, and catch hold of your feet. Keep your head on the mat.

2 Keeping hold of your feet, slowly lower your knees toward the floor as far as possible by extending your thighs.

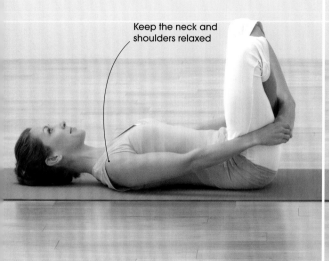

Keep the neck and shoulders relaxed

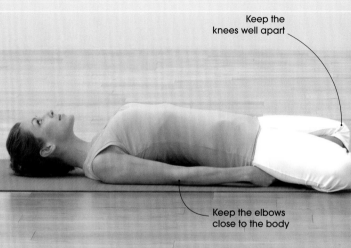

Keep the knees well apart

Keep the elbows close to the body

3 On an inhalation, firmly push on your elbows and move your hips up and forward, bringing your knees as close to the floor as possible. On another inhalation, lift your chest and bring the top of your head to the floor. Hold for up to 1 minute, then inhale, push your chest higher, and extend your neck. On an exhalation, lower your back to the floor and uncross your legs. Do the Neck Stretch (see p93), then relax for 1–2 minutes in Corpse Pose (see p188). Next time you practice this pose, cross your legs the opposite way.

Lift the chest

Keep the buttocks away from the feet

Do not put too much weight on your head

The weight is on the elbows

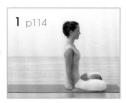

Start with

1 p114

Lotus Fish Advanced

2 Starting from Lotus final position, slowly lie back on the mat. Place your elbows close to your body and try to catch hold of your toes. Alternatively, place your hands on top of your hips.

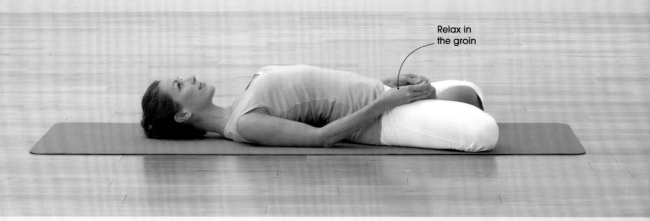

Relax in the groin

3 On an inhalation, bend your elbows and push your chest up. Slowly extend your neck until the top of your head is touching the floor. Hold for up to 1 minute, then inhale, push your chest higher, and extend your neck. On an exhalation, lower your back to the floor and uncross your legs. Do the Neck Stretch (see p93), then relax for 1–2 minutes in Corpse Pose (see p188). Next time you practice this pose, position your legs in Lotus in the opposite order.

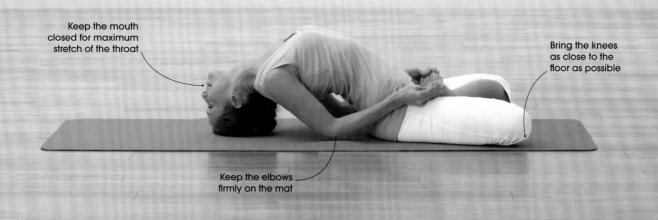

Keep the mouth closed for maximum stretch of the throat

Bring the knees as close to the floor as possible

Keep the elbows firmly on the mat

Forward Bend
Paschimotanasana

This pose can be very meditative. If you put equal emphasis on posture, breathing, and relaxation, it will balance the stimulation provided by the muscle stretches with your body's awareness of the pull of gravity. Practice Inclined Plane as a counterpose (see p100), then relax in Corpse Pose (see p188).

Benefits

PHYSICAL

- Stretches the posterior muscles completely from toes to neck.
- Reduces fat by putting pressure on the abdomen.
- Massages the liver, kidneys, and pancreas.
- Alleviates constipation.
- Relaxes the back muscles.
- Helps control diabetes.
- Calms and soothes the entire nervous system.

MENTAL

- This pose requires conscious control to align toes, knees, and neck correctly, and conscious letting go, by allowing gravity to pull the spine into the pose. Achieving control with detachment is a benefit that can be applied to daily life, as well as in the practice of meditation.

Forward Bend Beginner

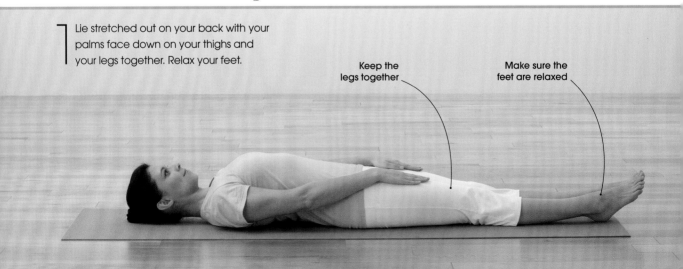

1 Lie stretched out on your back with your palms face down on your thighs and your legs together. Relax your feet.

Keep the legs together

Make sure the feet are relaxed

2 On an inhalation, sit up straight with your legs stretched out in front of you. Keep your head, neck, and back in a straight line.

3 On another inhalation, raise both arms straight up, stretching them as high as possible.

Align the arms with the ears

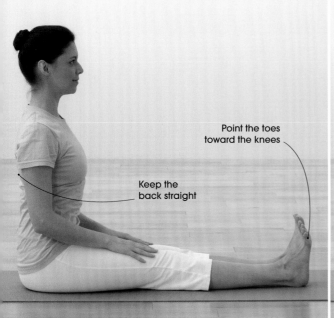

Point the toes toward the knees

Keep the back straight

4 Exhale and bend forward from the hips. Try to reach your calves or ankles with your hands. Repeat 3–4 times, each time holding the pose for a few breaths more. Either continue with Step 5 (see p98) or come back up on an inhalation. Next practice Inclined Plane (see p100), then relax in Corpse Pose (see p188).

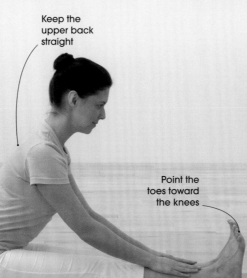

Keep the upper back straight

Point the toes toward the knees

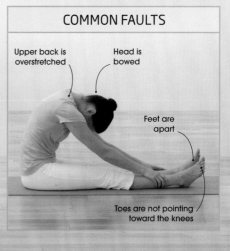

COMMON FAULTS

Upper back is overstretched

Head is bowed

Feet are apart

Toes are not pointing toward the knees

Forward Bend
Intermediate and Advanced

Progress in Forward Bend depends on how much you can lengthen the hamstring muscles at the back of your legs, which then allows the pelvis to tilt forward at the hip joint.

Start with

1 p96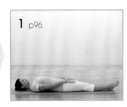

2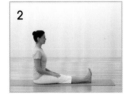

3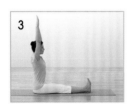

4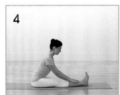

Intermediate

5 Starting from Forward Bend Step 4, if your hands reach your feet, take hold of your big toe in the Classical Foothold (see right).

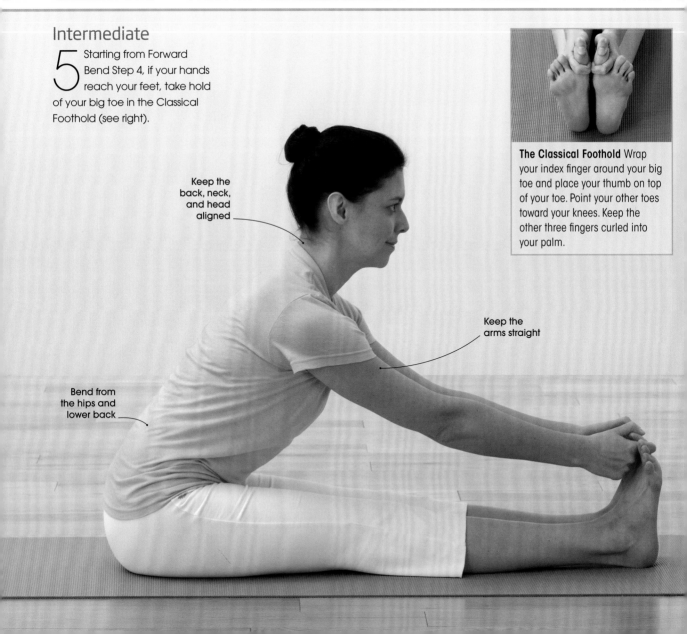

Keep the back, neck, and head aligned

Bend from the hips and lower back

Keep the arms straight

The Classical Foothold Wrap your index finger around your big toe and place your thumb on top of your toe. Point your other toes toward your knees. Keep the other three fingers curled into your palm.

6 On an exhalation, stretch your spine farther forward. Bend your elbows to help you stretch your spine. Repeat 3–4 times, each time holding the pose for a few breaths more. Either continue with Step 7 or come back up on an inhalation, then practice Inclined Plane (see pp100–101), and relax in Corpse Pose (see p191).

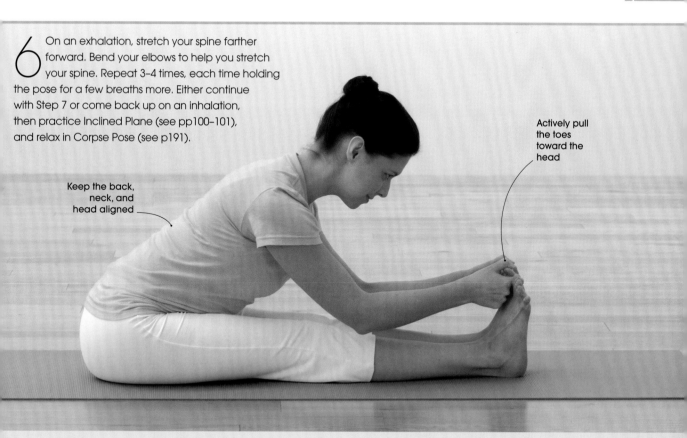

Keep the back, neck, and head aligned

Actively pull the toes toward the head

Advanced

7 If you are able to stretch forward, come into the full pose. On an exhalation, bend farther forward until your elbows touch the mat and your forehead is resting on your legs. Hold for 1–5 minutes, then come back up on an inhalation. Next, practice Inclined Plane (see pp100–101), then relax with slow abdominal breathing (see p46) for 1–2 minutes in Corpse Pose (see p188).

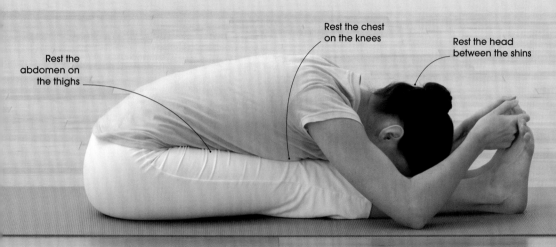

Rest the abdomen on the thighs

Rest the chest on the knees

Rest the head between the shins

Inclined Plane

All Levels

When you have practiced Forward Bend (see pp96-99), you should practice Inclined Plane as the counterpose. It will help to strengthen the muscles of your arms, legs, and back.

1 Sit with your legs stretched straight in front of you and place your hands about 12 in (30 cm) behind you on the mat. Drop your head backward, keeping your neck and throat relaxed. Rest on your hands.

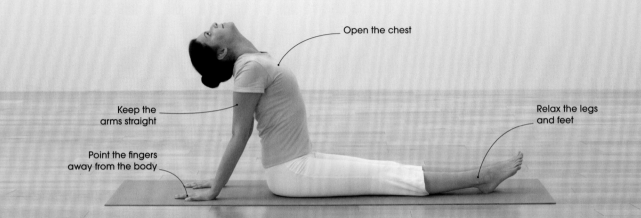

Open the chest

Keep the arms straight

Relax the legs and feet

Point the fingers away from the body

2 Inhale and lift your hips as high as possible. Hold your breath as you gently push your feet into the floor. Exhale and return to Step 1. Repeat twice more. Once you are accustomed to the pose, try to hold it, breathing rhythmically, for up to 30 seconds. Come down by bringing your hips back to the floor, then relax in Corpse Pose (see p188).

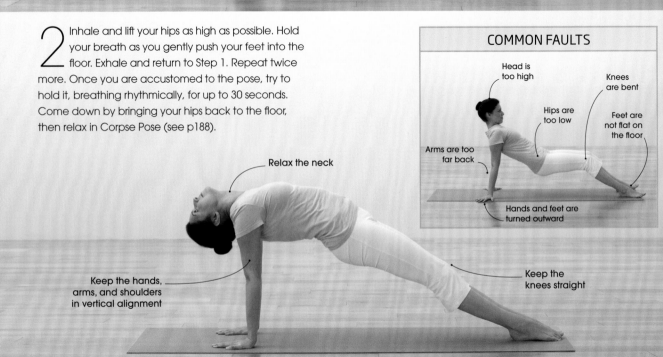

Relax the neck

Keep the hands, arms, and shoulders in vertical alignment

Keep the knees straight

COMMON FAULTS

Head is too high

Knees are bent

Hips are too low

Feet are not flat on the floor

Arms are too far back

Hands and feet are turned outward

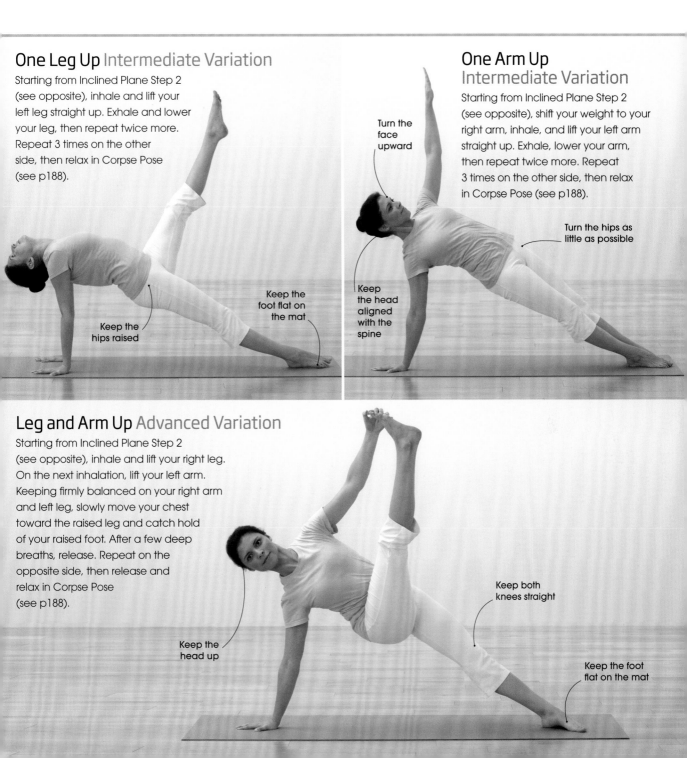

One Leg Up Intermediate Variation

Starting from Inclined Plane Step 2
(see opposite), inhale and lift your
left leg straight up. Exhale and lower
your leg, then repeat twice more.
Repeat 3 times on the other
side, then relax in Corpse Pose
(see p188).

Keep the foot flat on the mat

Keep the hips raised

One Arm Up
Intermediate Variation

Starting from Inclined Plane Step 2
(see opposite), shift your weight to your
right arm, inhale, and lift your left arm
straight up. Exhale, lower your arm,
then repeat twice more. Repeat
3 times on the other side, then relax
in Corpse Pose (see p188).

Turn the face upward

Turn the hips as little as possible

Keep the head aligned with the spine

Leg and Arm Up Advanced Variation

Starting from Inclined Plane Step 2
(see opposite), inhale and lift your right leg.
On the next inhalation, lift your left arm.
Keeping firmly balanced on your right arm
and left leg, slowly move your chest
toward the raised leg and catch hold
of your raised foot. After a few deep
breaths, release. Repeat on the
opposite side, then release and
relax in Corpse Pose
(see p188).

Keep the head up

Keep both knees straight

Keep the foot flat on the mat

Forward Bend
Variations

When practicing Forward Bend variations, practice the counterpose–Inclined Plane (see p100)–between each variation and after you practice your last variation.

Single Leg Forward Bend Beginner

1 Sit with your legs stretched out in front of you, then bend your right knee and place the sole of your right foot against your left thigh. Inhale and raise your arms over your head.

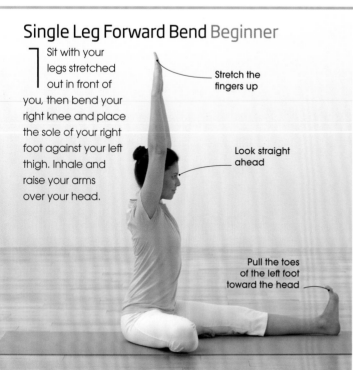

Stretch the fingers up

Look straight ahead

Pull the toes of the left foot toward the head

2 Exhale, bend from the waist over your left leg, and place your hands on your leg, ankle, or foot. With each exhalation, let your spine move forward. Aim to rest your abdomen on your thigh, your chest on your knee, and your head on your shin. Hold the pose for 1–3 minutes. Release and repeat on the opposite side. Practice Inclined Plane (see p100), then relax in Corpse Pose (see p188).

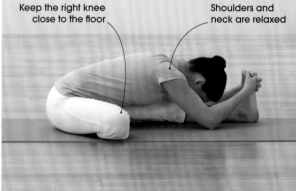

Keep the right knee close to the floor

Shoulders and neck are relaxed

Butterfly Beginner

1 Sit with your legs stretched out in front of you, then bend your knees, take hold of your feet, and bring them close to your body.

Make sure the back, neck, and head are aligned

Keep the soles of the feet together

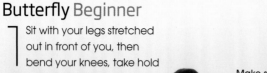
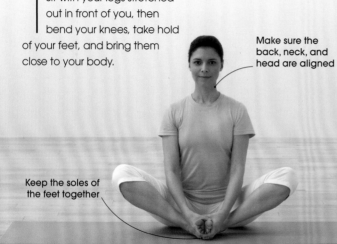

2 Rhythmically push your knees down toward the floor, then release so they come back up. Repeat 10–20 times. Release and relax in Corpse Pose (see p188).

Keep the chest open

Aim to reach the floor with your knees

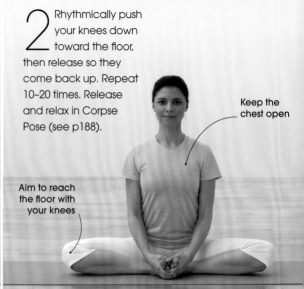

Half Lotus Forward Bend Intermediate

1 Sit with your legs stretched out in front of you, then bend your left knee and take your left foot on top of your right thigh, close to your hips. This is Half Lotus. Inhale and raise your arms over your head. If your left knee does not rest on the floor, you should practice only Single Leg Forward Bend (see opposite).

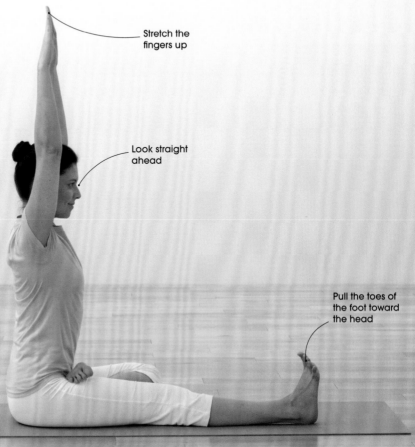

Stretch the fingers up

Look straight ahead

Pull the toes of the foot toward the head

2 With an exhalation, bend from the waist over your right leg and reach forward. Place your hands on your leg or ankle, or hold onto your foot. With each exhalation, allow your spine to move forward more. Hold the pose for 1–3 minutes. Release and repeat on the opposite side. Practice Inclined Plane (see p100), then relax in Corpse Pose (see p188).

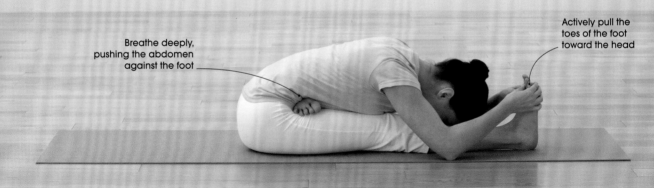

Breathe deeply, pushing the abdomen against the foot

Actively pull the toes of the foot toward the head

Forward Bend
Variations (continued)

These Forward Bend variations work on the flexion, abduction, and external rotation of the hip joints. They will make everyday sitting, standing, and walking much easier.

Forward Bend with Wide Legs
Intermediate

1 Sit with your legs as wide apart as possible and your feet pointing toward the ceiling. Inhale and lift your arms high over your head.

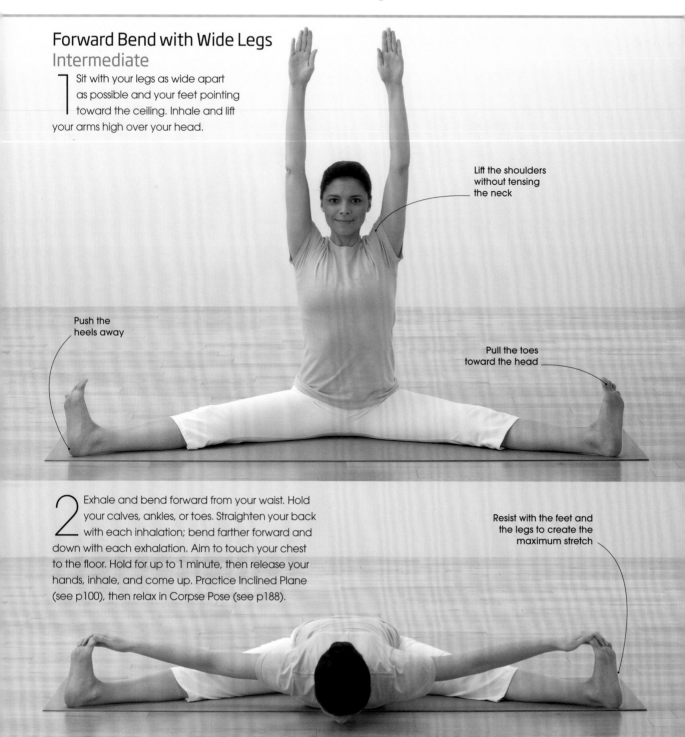

Lift the shoulders without tensing the neck

Push the heels away

Pull the toes toward the head

2 Exhale and bend forward from your waist. Hold your calves, ankles, or toes. Straighten your back with each inhalation; bend farther forward and down with each exhalation. Aim to touch your chest to the floor. Hold for up to 1 minute, then release your hands, inhale, and come up. Practice Inclined Plane (see p100), then relax in Corpse Pose (see p188).

Resist with the feet and the legs to create the maximum stretch

Start with

1 p103

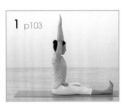

Bound Half Lotus Forward Bend Advanced

2 Starting from Half Lotus Forward Bend Step 1, bring your left arm behind your back and hold your left foot. Exhale, bend from the waist, and reach forward to hold the toes of your right foot. Hold the pose for up to 1 minute. Release and repeat on the opposite side. Practice Inclined Plane (see p100), then relax in Corpse Pose (see p188).

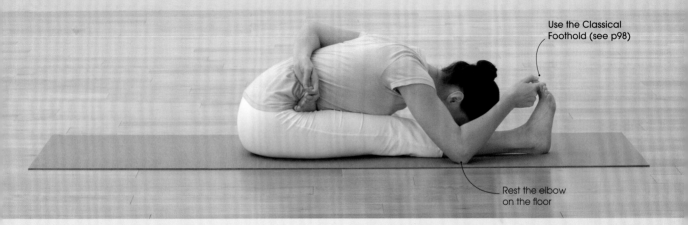

Use the Classical Foothold (see p98)

Rest the elbow on the floor

Straight Arm Forward Bend Advanced

1 Sitting with your legs outstretched, inhale, raise your arms, then exhale and bend forward. Put your hands in Prayer Position (see p50) and place your hands, wrists, or forearms on your toes. Hold for up to 1 minute, then release. Practice Inclined Plane (see p100), then relax in Corpse Pose (see p188).

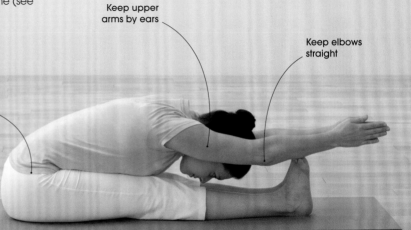

Keep upper arms by ears

Keep elbows straight

Bend forward from the hip joint

Forward Bend
Variations (continued)

These Forward Bend variations are good examples of how asanas prepare you for the meditative sitting poses (see p203). They help you to gain the necessary flexibility, strength, and balance.

Tortoise Advanced

1 Sit with legs apart, knees bent, and feet flat on the floor, as close to your body as possible. Bend forward and place your arms under your bent knees, reaching as far back as possible.

2 With an exhalation, bend forward from the waist until your chin, forehead, or chest touches the floor. Push your heels forward and straighten your knees as much as possible. Hold, breathing rhythmically, for up to 1 minute, then slide your legs closer to you until you can take your arms out from underneath your knees. Practice Inclined Plane (see p100), then relax in Corpse Pose (see p188).

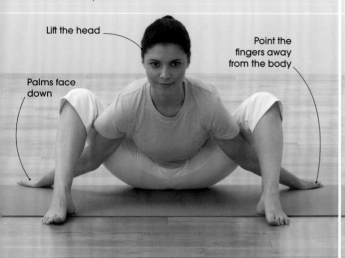

Lift the head

Point the fingers away from the body

Palms face down

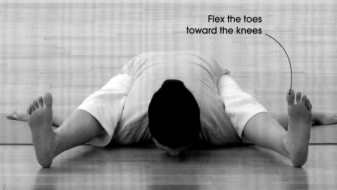

Flex the toes toward the knees

Seated One Leg Raise Advanced

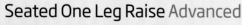

Sit with your legs stretched out in front of you, then bend your right leg and place your right foot in front of your body. Bend forward, reach for your left leg, and pull it straight up, holding onto your calf, ankle, or toes. Hold, breathing rhythmically, for up to 1 minute. Release and repeat on the opposite side. Practice Inclined Plane (see p100), then relax in Corpse Pose (see p188).

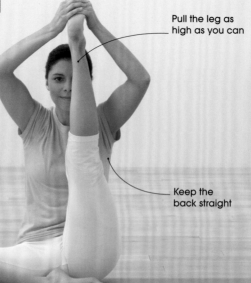

Pull the leg as high as you can

Keep the back straight

Start with

1 p102

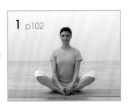

Seated Two Leg Raise Advanced

2 Before beginning, make sure there is enough space behind you in case you lose your balance and roll backward. Starting from Butterfly Step 1, inhale and pull both legs straight up in front of you. Clasp your calves, ankles, or toes. Hold, breathing rhythmically, for 30 seconds, then release. Practice Inclined Plane (see p100), then relax in Corpse Pose (see p188).

Use the arms to extend the back higher

Sit forward on the buttocks, as far from the lower back as possible

Lateral Bend with Twist Advanced

Sit with legs apart, feet pointing upward. Place your right foot in front of your groin or against your left thigh. Inhale, stretch both arms up, and twist to the right. Exhale and bend sideways. Catch your big left toe in the Classical Foothold (see p98) and place your right hand on the outside of your left foot. Hold, breathing rhythmically, for up to 1 minute. Release and repeat on the opposite side. Practice Inclined Plane (see p100), then relax in Corpse Pose (see p188).

Turn the head to face forward

Keep both buttocks on the mat

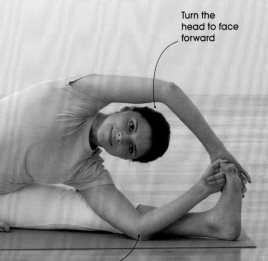

Place the elbow on the knee or on the floor

One Foot to Head
All Levels

Try these challenging poses according to your level of ability. Rest afterward in Corpse Pose (see p188) so the muscles of your pelvis and lower back can relax completely.

Beginner

1 Starting from a sitting position, bring your left foot close to your body. Lift your right leg and cradle your right knee and foot. With a rhythmical exhalation and inhalation, gently rock to and fro to twist the spine and open the hip joint. Repeat 4 times, then repeat on the opposite side. Continue with Step 2 or relax in Corpse Pose (see p188).

Keep the back straight

Keep the calf parallel to the floor

Intermediate

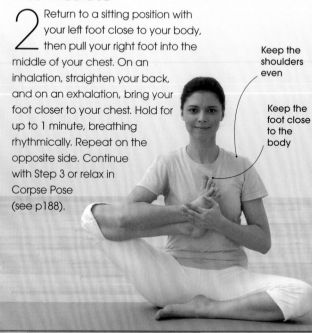

2 Return to a sitting position with your left foot close to your body, then pull your right foot into the middle of your chest. On an inhalation, straighten your back, and on an exhalation, bring your foot closer to your chest. Hold for up to 1 minute, breathing rhythmically. Repeat on the opposite side. Continue with Step 3 or relax in Corpse Pose (see p188).

Keep the shoulders even

Keep the foot close to the body

Advanced

3 Return to a sitting position with your left foot close to your body. Use both hands to pull your right knee over your right shoulder. Breathing deeply, hold for up to 1 minute, then repeat on the opposite side.

Take the knee over the shoulder

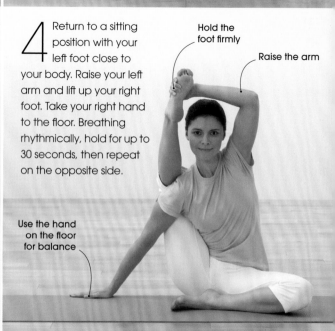

4 Return to a sitting position with your left foot close to your body. Raise your left arm and lift up your right foot. Take your right hand to the floor. Breathing rhythmically, hold for up to 30 seconds, then repeat on the opposite side.

Hold the foot firmly

Raise the arm

Use the hand on the floor for balance

5 To come into the full pose, return to a sitting position with your left foot close to your body. Bend your head forward and use your left hand to pull your right foot behind your head. Take your head back against your right foot and place your hands in Prayer Position (see p50) in front of your chest. Hold for a few rhythmical breaths, then release the pose by following Steps 4 and 3 in that order. Repeat with your head against your left foot, then relax in Corpse Pose (see p188).

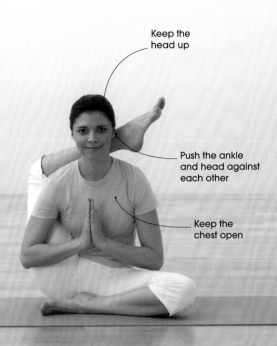

Keep the head up

Push the ankle and head against each other

Keep the chest open

Lying Down Leg Behind Head
Advanced variation

Starting from One Foot to Head Step 5 (see above), stretch out your left leg and slowly lie down on the mat, keeping your right foot behind your head and your hands in Prayer Position (see p50). Hold for a few rhythmical breaths, then take hold of your right foot with your right hand, and carefully release your right leg. Repeat on the opposite side, then relax in Corpse Pose (see p188).

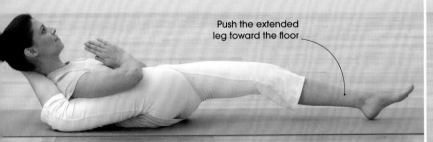

Push the extended leg toward the floor

Both Legs Behind Head
Advanced variation

Starting from Lying Down Leg Behind Head (see left), take your left foot behind your head. Lock your left foot with the right. Clasp your hands under your lower back. Hold for a few rhythmical breaths, then unlock your feet and roll out of the pose. Repeat on the opposite side, then relax in Corpse Pose (see p188).

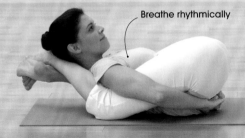

Breathe rhythmically

Shooting Bow
Advanced

These variations will help you to improve your Forward Bend (see pp96-99). Whenever you practice Shooting Bow, return to Forward Bend and then practice Inclined Plane (see p100) as a counterpose.

Start with

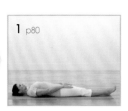 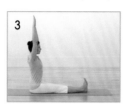 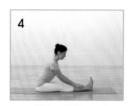 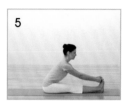

1 p80

2

3

4

5

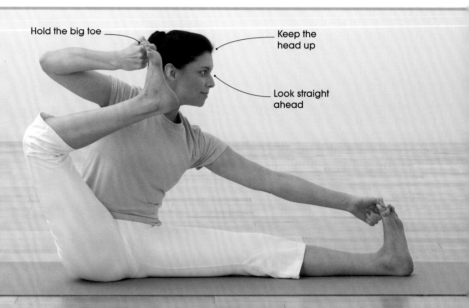

6 Starting from Forward Bend Step 5, inhale and bend your right knee, pulling your right foot back and up as close to your right ear as possible. Keep your raised elbow as high as possible. After a few breaths, release your foot, then repeat on the opposite side. Return to Forward Bend Step 5, then practice Inclined Plane (see p100). Finally, relax in Corpse Pose (see p188).

Hold the big toe

Keep the head up

Look straight ahead

Diagonal Shooting Bow Variation

Starting from Forward Bend Step 5, take your left arm on top of your right so each hand is holding the opposite foot. Inhale and pull your left foot toward your right ear. After a few breaths, release your leg, then repeat, crossing your arms the other way and pulling your right foot toward your left ear. Return to Forward Bend Step 5, then practice Inclined Plane (see p100). Finally, relax in Corpse Pose (see p188).

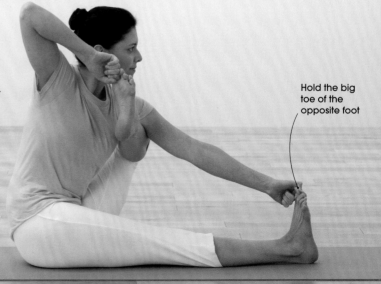

Hold the big toe of the opposite foot

"Asanas give strength. Pranayama gives lightness of body. Meditation gives perception of the Self and leads to freedom or final beatitude." Swami Sivananda

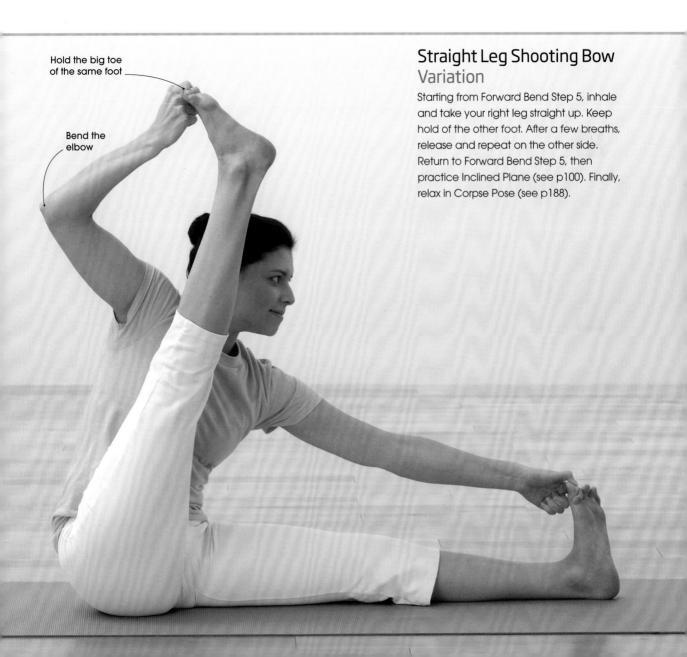

Hold the big toe of the same foot

Bend the elbow

Straight Leg Shooting Bow
Variation

Starting from Forward Bend Step 5, inhale and take your right leg straight up. Keep hold of the other foot. After a few breaths, release and repeat on the other side. Return to Forward Bend Step 5, then practice Inclined Plane (see p100). Finally, relax in Corpse Pose (see p188).

Splits
Advanced

Splits and its variations progressively open up the hip and shoulder joints, as well as the solar plexus area in the abdomen. This allows plenty of prana (vital energy, see p178) to flow through the body.

Splits

Kneel down and take your left leg forward. Breathe slowly as you place your hands either side of your body to help you balance, then straighten your right leg behind and push your left heel farther away to deepen the split. If you are flexible enough to sit down, take your hands into Prayer Position (see p50) in front of your chest. Hold for a few breaths then, pressing your hands against the mat, release the pose by bending both legs. Repeat on the other side, then relax in Corpse Pose (see p188).

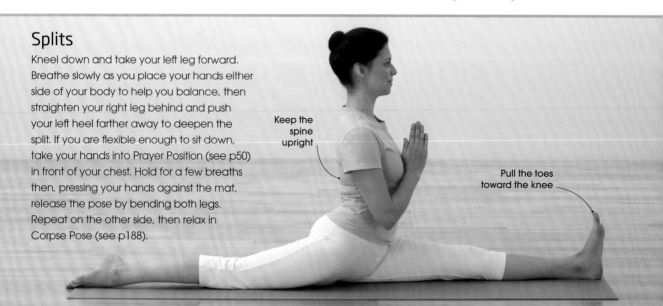

Keep the spine upright

Pull the toes toward the knee

Crescent Splits Variation

1 Starting from Splits (see above), with an inhalation, take your arms straight up alongside your ears. Keep your balance by using rhythmical breathing and looking at a point in front of you.

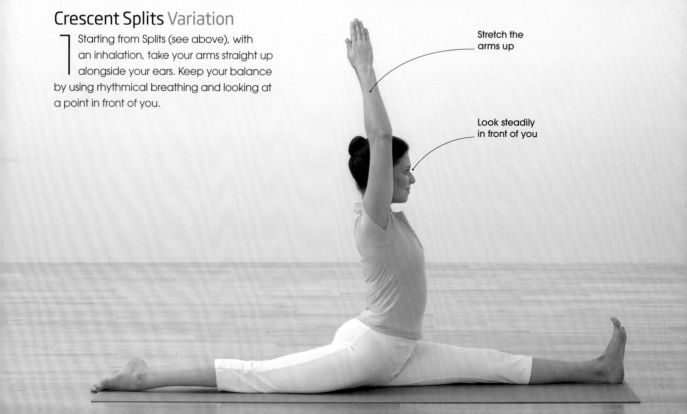

Stretch the arms up

Look steadily in front of you

2 Still keeping your arms straight, inhale and arch your upper body backward. Hold for a few breaths, then bring your arms down and release the pose as for Splits (see opposite). Repeat on the other side, release, then relax in Corpse Pose (see p188).

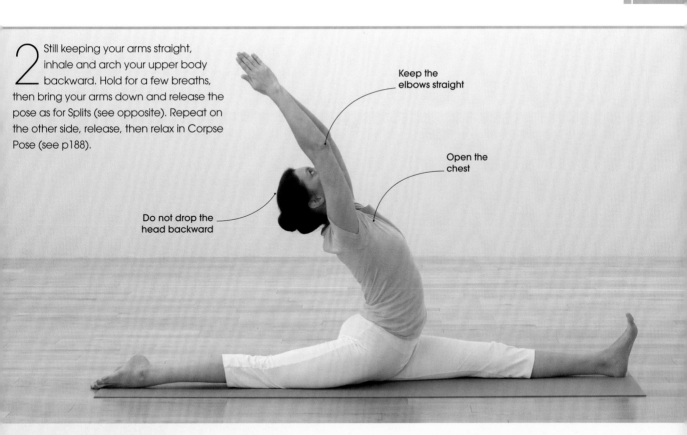

Keep the elbows straight

Open the chest

Do not drop the head backward

Pigeon Splits Variation

Starting from Crescent Splits Step 2 (see above), breathe rhythmically as you bend your right knee and catch hold of your right foot with both hands. Hold for a few breaths, then release your hold on your foot and release the pose as for Splits (see opposite). Repeat on the other side, release, then relax in Corpse Pose (see p188).

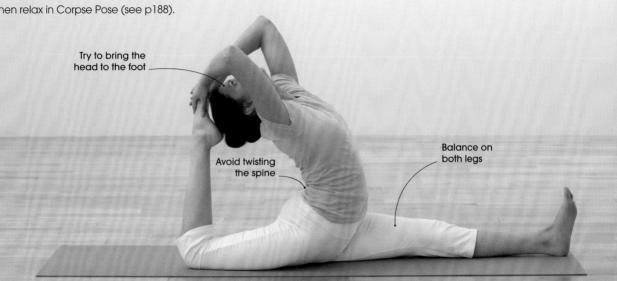

Try to bring the head to the foot

Avoid twisting the spine

Balance on both legs

Lotus
Advanced

Lotus gives you a very stable base so you can keep your back aligned without much effort. The various triangular shapes that your body makes in this pose allow a free flow of prana (see p178).

1 Sit cross-legged, then lift your left foot on top of your right thigh, taking the foot as close to your right hip as possible. If necessary, you can place a small pillow under your sitting bones. Breathe slowly and meditatively.

2 Lift your right foot on top of your left thigh and rest your hands, palms face upward, on your knees in Chin Mudra position (see p204). Hold the pose, breathing slowly and meditatively, for 1 minute, then release first the right foot, then the left. Repeat, placing first your right foot on your left thigh and then your left foot on your right thigh. Hold for 1 minute, then release and relax in Corpse Pose (see p188).

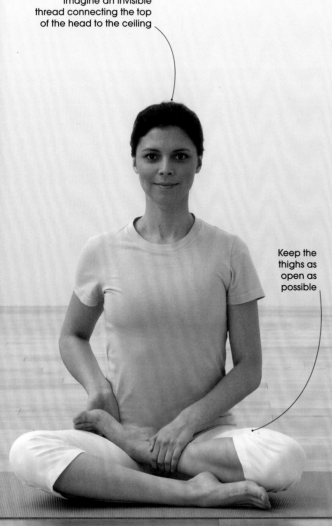

Imagine an invisible thread connecting the top of the head to the ceiling

Keep the thighs as open as possible

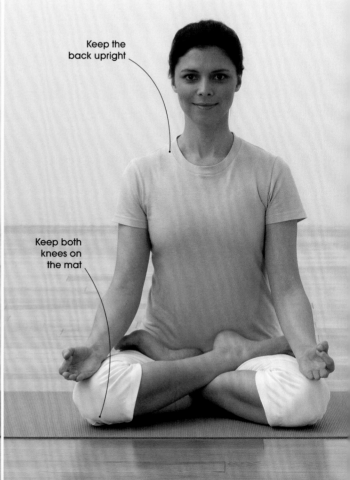

Keep the back upright

Keep both knees on the mat

Lotus Balance Variation

Starting from Lotus Step 2 (see opposite), lie on your back. Place your arms under your body with your palms under your buttocks. Inhale, contract your abdominal muscles, and raise first your head and chest, then your knees. Hold, breathing deeply, for up to 30 seconds, then bring your knees down and carefully remove your arms and lie back down. Repeat with your legs folded the other way, then release and relax in Corpse Pose (see p188).

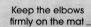

Bring the head forward

Keep the elbows firmly on the mat

Lying Fish Variation

Starting from Lotus Step 2 (see opposite), lie on your abdomen. Fold your arms and rest your forehead on them. Hold, breathing very slowly and quietly, for up to 1 minute, then come out of the pose by pushing on your elbows and swinging your legs forward to return to Lotus Step 2. Unfold your legs, then repeat with your legs folded the other way. Release and relax in Child's Pose (see p191).

Keep the thighs as flat as possible

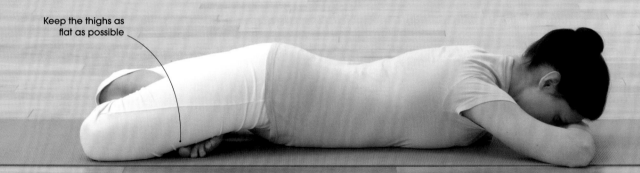

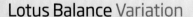

6 Cobra
Bujangasana

Like a cobra with its hood raised, in Bhujangasana you arch your head and trunk upward. Backward bending against the pull of gravity is the most efficient way to develop a strong back. After Cobra you can either relax on your abdomen (see p190) or stretch back into Child's Pose (see p191).

Benefits

PHYSICAL
- Tones the deep and superficial muscles of the back.
- Increases the blood supply to the ligaments of the spine and the vertebrae.
- Removes any tension from overworked back muscles.
- Relieves kyphosis—exaggerated thoracic curvature (see p29).
- Massages the abdominal organs.
- Combats constipation.
- Tones the ovaries and uterus and alleviates menstrual problems.

MENTAL
- By requiring you to focus fully on contracting the muscles in your neck and upper back, Cobra helps to develop your powers of concentration.

Cobra Beginner and Intermediate

Beginner

1 Lie on your abdomen, keeping your legs straight and your toes together. Point your toes, take your forehead to the mat, and bring your hands alongside your chest, palms face down.

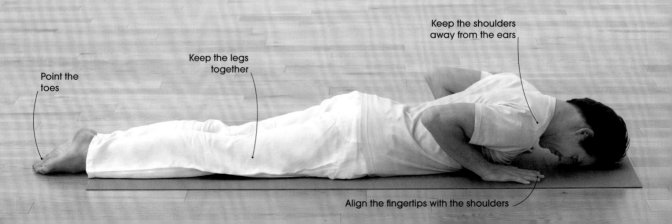

Point the toes

Keep the legs together

Keep the shoulders away from the ears

Align the fingertips with the shoulders

2 On an inhalation, take your hands off the floor, and lift your head, shoulders, and upper back. Take your elbows behind your back, close to your body. Hold for 5 deep breaths, then slowly lower your body back to the floor. Repeat 3 times. Continue with Step 3 or relax for a few breaths on your abdomen (see p190) or in Child's Pose (see p191).

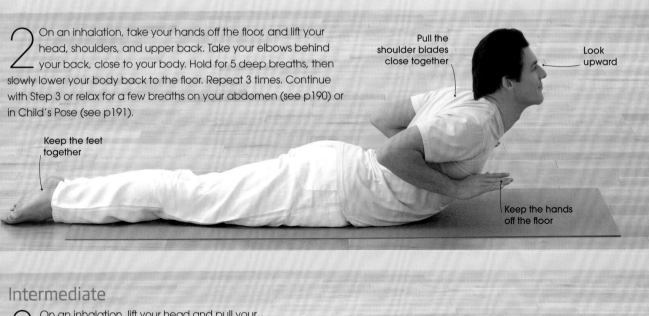

Pull the shoulder blades close together

Look upward

Keep the feet together

Keep the hands off the floor

Intermediate

3 On an inhalation, lift your head and pull your shoulder blades in toward each other. Keep your chest on the floor.

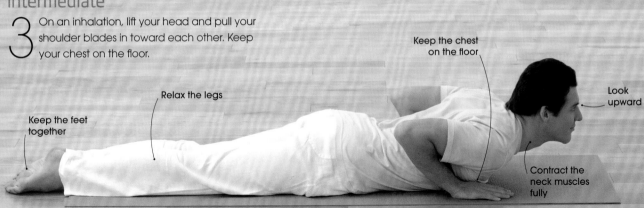

Keep the chest on the floor

Look upward

Relax the legs

Keep the feet together

Contract the neck muscles fully

4 On the next inhalation, lift your head further and raise your chest off the floor. Keep pulling your shoulder blades together. Hold for up to 30 seconds, then slowly lower your body back to the floor. Repeat, then either continue with Step 5 (see p118) or relax for a few breaths on your abdomen (see p190) or in Child's Pose (see p191).

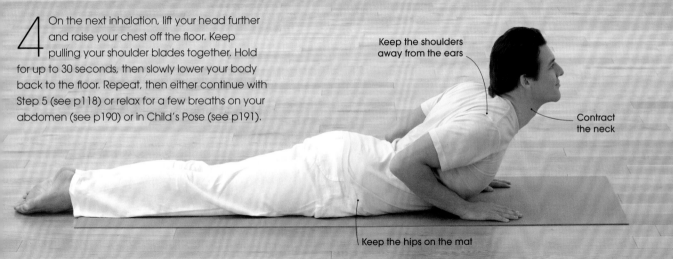

Keep the shoulders away from the ears

Contract the neck

Keep the hips on the mat

Cobra
Advanced

Working at a desk encourages rounded shoulders and a collapsed chest, which impairs breathing and depresses your mood. Daily practice of Cobra, at any level, can help to rectify these problems.

Start with

1 p116

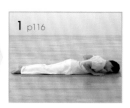

2

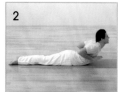

3

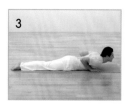

4

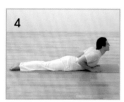

5 To come into the full pose, start from Cobra Step 4. On an inhalation, arch your head, neck, and upper back as much as possible. Keep your legs together and make sure that your shoulder blades are pulled backward and away from your ears. Hold for up to 1 minute, then lower your body back to the floor. Take a few deep breaths, then repeat. Relax on your abdomen (see p190) for a few breaths, or relax in Child's Pose (see p191).

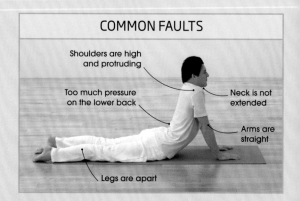

COMMON FAULTS

Shoulders are high and protruding

Neck is not extended

Too much pressure on the lower back

Arms are straight

Legs are apart

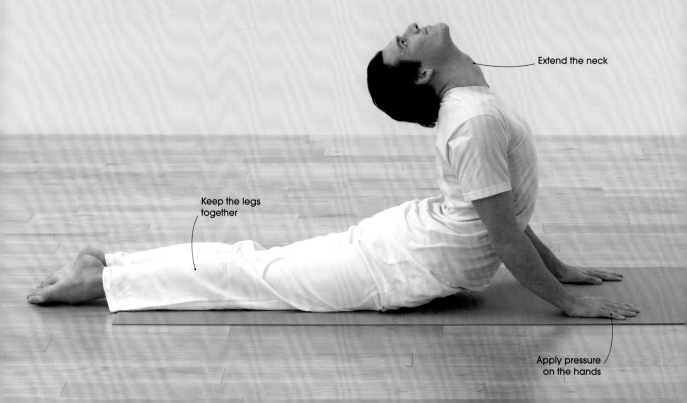

Extend the neck

Keep the legs together

Apply pressure on the hands

Start with

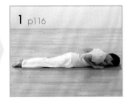

1 p116

Hands Clasped Intermediate Variation

2 Starting from Cobra Step 1, take your arms behind your back, straighten them, and clasp your hands together.

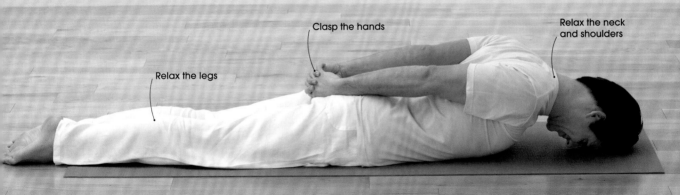

Clasp the hands

Relax the neck and shoulders

Relax the legs

3 With an inhalation, lift your head, arms, and chest off the floor. Hold for up to 30 seconds, then lower your body back to the floor. Take a few deep breaths, then repeat. Relax on your abdomen (see p190) for a few breaths, or relax in Child's Pose (see p191).

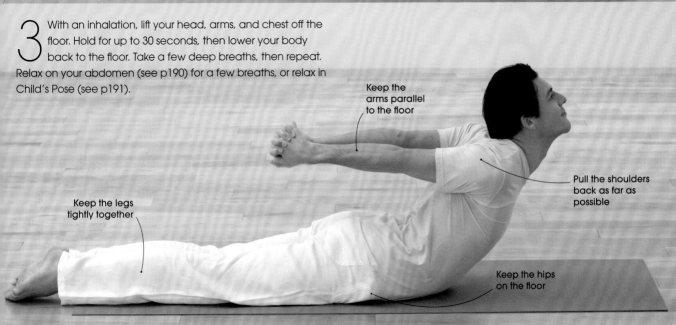

Keep the arms parallel to the floor

Pull the shoulders back as far as possible

Keep the legs tightly together

Keep the hips on the floor

Cobra
Variations (continued)

King Cobra majestically combines contraction of your neck and of the muscles of your upper back with a complete backward bend of your spine. An added benefit is an increase in your lung capacity.

Start with

1 p116

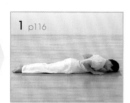

King Cobra Advanced

2 Starting from Cobra Step 1, place your hands next to the lower part of your rib cage, and bend your legs up. Keep your legs apart with your feet touching each other.

Touch the feet together

Relax the shoulders and neck

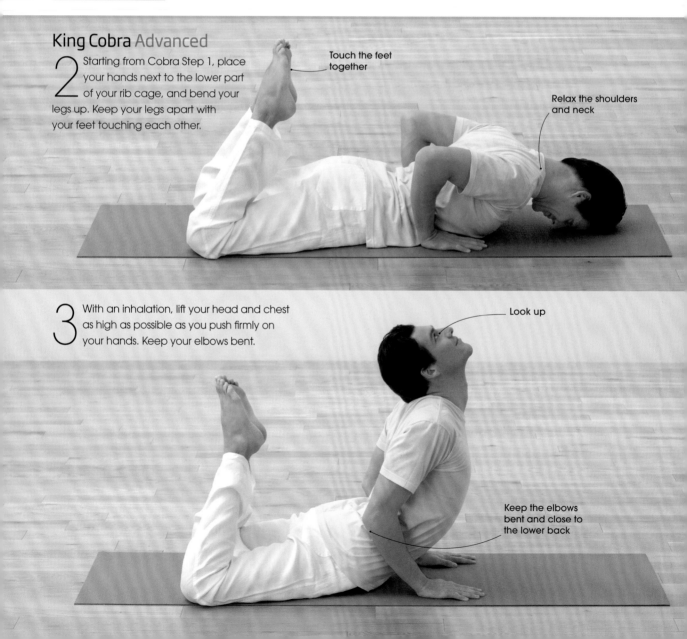

3 With an inhalation, lift your head and chest as high as possible as you push firmly on your hands. Keep your elbows bent.

Look up

Keep the elbows bent and close to the lower back

4 With another inhalation, lift your head and chest even higher. Straighten your arms completely and bring your feet to your head. Hold for up to 30 seconds, then take your feet from your head, and lower your body back to the floor. Take a few deep breaths, then repeat. Relax on your abdomen (see p190) for a few breaths, or relax in Child's Pose (see p191).

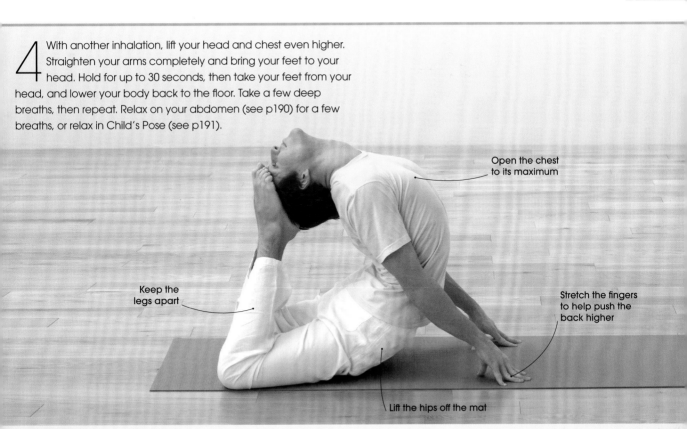

Open the chest to its maximum

Keep the legs apart

Stretch the fingers to help push the back higher

Lift the hips off the mat

King Cobra Knee Hold Advanced

Starting from King Cobra Step 4 (see above), lift one hand and catch your knee. Find your balance, then catch your other knee with the other hand. Hold for a few breaths, replace your hands in front of you, as in King Cobra Step 4, then lower your body back to the floor. Take a few deep breaths, then repeat. Relax on your abdomen (see p190) for a few breaths, or relax in Child's Pose (see p191).

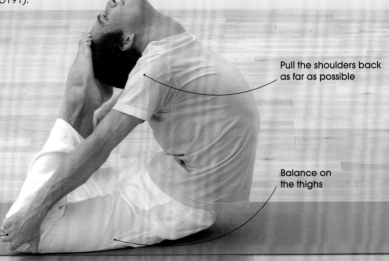

Pull the shoulders back as far as possible

Balance on the thighs

Hold the knees firmly

7 Locust
Salabhasana

Unlike the other asanas, which are done slowly, you achieve Locust with a single powerful muscle contraction, similar to a locust jumping. This brings together thought, breath, movement, and prana—vital energy (see p178). After Locust, stretch back into Child's Pose (see p191) or relax on your front (see p190).

Benefits

PHYSICAL

• Strengthens the muscles of the arms, shoulders, abdomen, lower back, thighs, and legs.

• Tones the liver, pancreas, and kidneys.

• Improves the appetite.

• Relieves constipation.

MENTAL

• Of all the asanas, this pose is the one that works most on developing will power. According to Swami Vishnudevananda, exercising will power makes one's thoughts pure and powerful and is the main goal of the practice of asanas. Strong will power also lifts your energy levels from inertia (tamas, see p212) to harmony (satva, see p212).

Locust All Levels

Beginner

1 Lie on your abdomen with your legs outstretched, heels together, arms under your body, and chin forward on the mat. Place your hands in one of the hand positions (see right), depending on which you find most comfortable. Hand position A is the classical position for this pose.

Hand position A
Interlock the fingers and keep the thumbs together.

Hand position B
Clench the fists and keep the thumbs together.

Keep the elbows close together

Point the toes

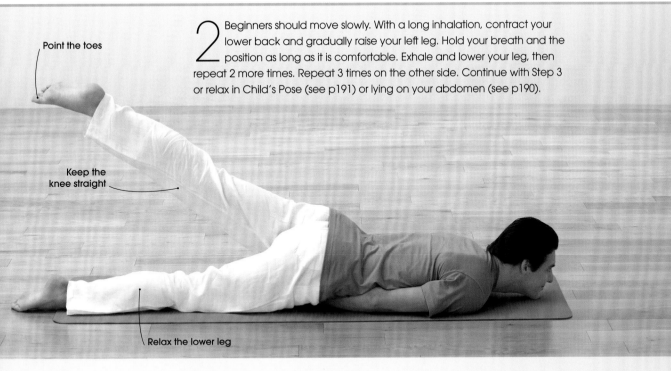

Point the toes

Keep the
knee straight

Relax the lower leg

2 Beginners should move slowly. With a long inhalation, contract your lower back and gradually raise your left leg. Hold your breath and the position as long as it is comfortable. Exhale and lower your leg, then repeat 2 more times. Repeat 3 times on the other side. Continue with Step 3 or relax in Child's Pose (see p191) or lying on your abdomen (see p190).

Intermediate and Advanced

3 To come into the full pose, on a quick, strong inhalation, contract your lower back, push on your arms, and swing both legs up as high as possible. Hold your breath as long as is comfortable, then exhale and lower your legs. Repeat 2 more times, then relax in Child's Pose (see p191) or lying on your abdomen (see p190).

Point the toes

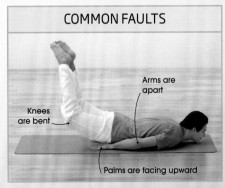

COMMON FAULTS

Arms are
apart

Knees
are bent

Palms are facing upward

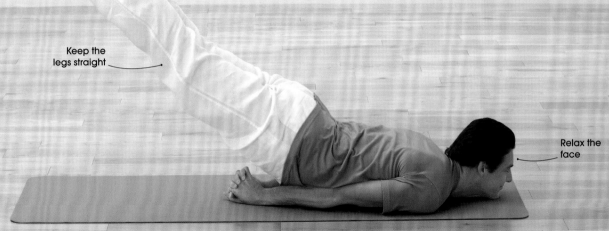

Keep the
legs straight

Relax the
face

Locust
Variations

The Boat variations are very efficient. You contract your back muscles strongly without putting much pressure on your vertebrae. For maximum benefit, go into and come out of these poses very slowly.

Boat Beginner

1 Lie face down on the mat with your arms stretched out in front of you and your feet extended behind. Rest your forehead on the floor and breathe deeply in your abdomen. Exhale completely.

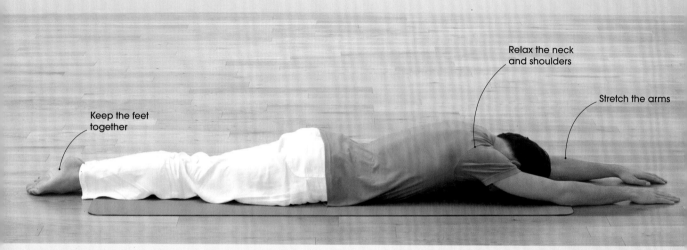

Keep the feet together

Relax the neck and shoulders

Stretch the arms

2 On an inhalation, simultaneously lift both your arms and legs as high as possible. You may hold your breath or take a few deep breaths in your abdomen. Exhale and release. Repeat up to 3 times, then relax in Child's Pose (see p191) or lying on your abdomen (see p190).

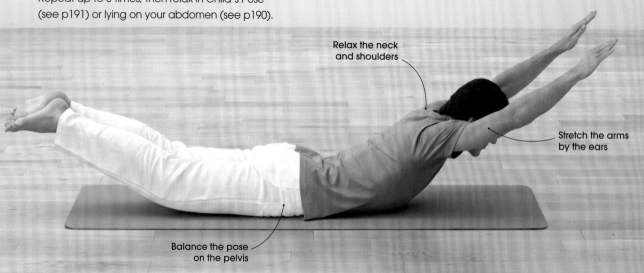

Relax the neck and shoulders

Stretch the arms by the ears

Balance the pose on the pelvis

Boat with Interlock Advanced

1 Lie face down on the mat with your feet extended behind you and your forehead on the floor. Take your arms behind your back and hold onto your elbows. Exhale completely.

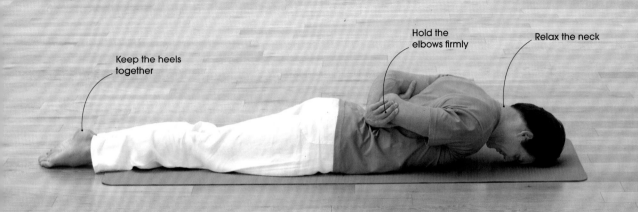

Keep the heels together

Hold the elbows firmly

Relax the neck

2 On an inhalation, lift your legs, head, and chest as high as possible. You may hold your breath or take a few deep breaths. Exhale and release. Repeat up to 3 times, then relax in Child's Pose (see p191) or lying on your abdomen (see p190).

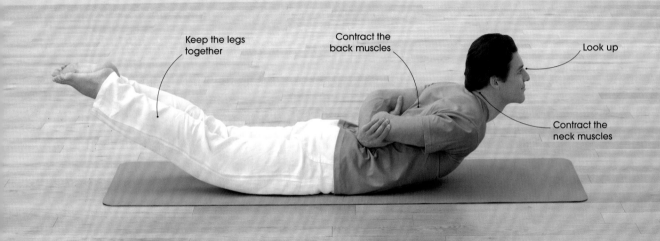

Keep the legs together

Contract the back muscles

Look up

Contract the neck muscles

Locust
Variations (continued)

These Locust variations require regular practice. This will enable you to contract your lower back muscles fast and strongly enough to bring your legs up higher than in Intermediate Locust.

Start with

1 p122

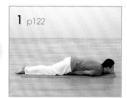

2

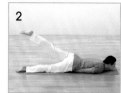

3

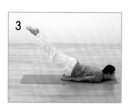

High Legs Advanced

3 Starting from Locust Step 3, inhale and swing your legs up as quickly as you can, adding a strong push with your arms against the floor. Hold for a few breaths, then come out of the pose by slowly releasing the contraction of your back and resisting with your arms. Take a few deep breaths, then repeat. Continue with Feet to Head (see right) or relax in Child's Pose (see p191) or lying on your abdomen (see p190).

Keep the legs straight

Push the hands and arms firmly into the mat

Feet to Head Advanced

Starting from High Legs (see left), focus on taking long exhalations as you bend your knees and lower your feet as close to your head as possible. Hold for a few breaths, then come out of the pose by slowly releasing the contraction of your back and resisting with your arms. Take a few deep breaths, then repeat. Relax in Child's Pose (see p191) or lying on your abdomen (see p190).

Keep the legs apart

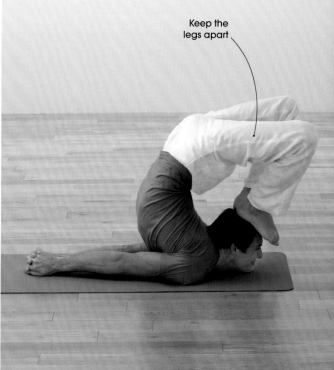

Locust in Lotus Advanced

1 Start by sitting in Lotus (see p114). Take a few complete yogic breaths (see p181).

2 Leaning forward, take your hands onto the floor in front of you and come up onto your knees. Walk your hands forward until your hands are beneath your shoulders. Breathe slowly and rhythmically.

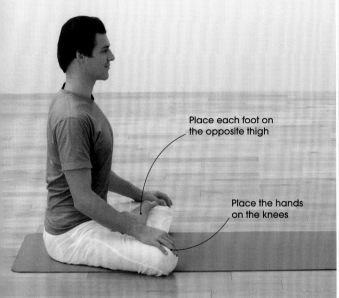

Place each foot on the opposite thigh

Place the hands on the knees

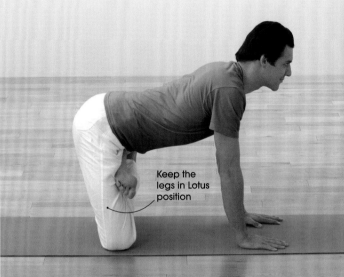

Keep the legs in Lotus position

3 Without releasing your legs, gently lower yourself into a lying position with your arms under your body. Place your hands in one of the hand positions shown on p122, whichever is the most comfortable. Exhale completely.

4 Inhale and swing your legs up as quickly and as high as possible. Use the strength of your arms and of your lower back to come up. Hold the pose for a few breaths, then come out by slowly releasing the contraction of your back and resisting with your arms. Repeat, crossing your legs the other way. Relax in Child's Pose (see p191) or lying on your abdomen (see p190).

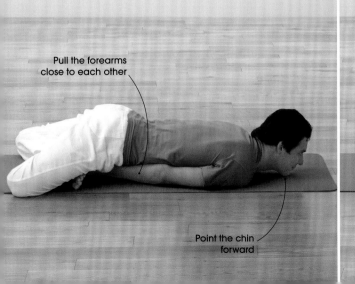

Pull the forearms close to each other

Point the chin forward

Strongly push the hands and arms against the mat

Camel
Beginner and Intermediate

Camel is a more passive backward bend that stretches your chest and throat muscles. It also requires you to balance, which strengthens your hamstrings and the muscles of your buttocks.

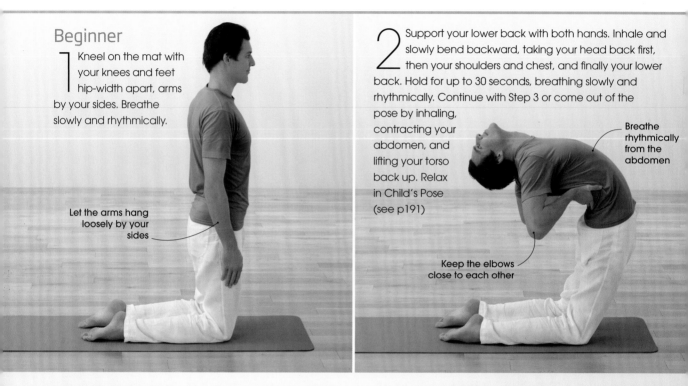

Beginner

1 Kneel on the mat with your knees and feet hip-width apart, arms by your sides. Breathe slowly and rhythmically.

Let the arms hang loosely by your sides

2 Support your lower back with both hands. Inhale and slowly bend backward, taking your head back first, then your shoulders and chest, and finally your lower back. Hold for up to 30 seconds, breathing slowly and rhythmically. Continue with Step 3 or come out of the pose by inhaling, contracting your abdomen, and lifting your torso back up. Relax in Child's Pose (see p191)

Breathe rhythmically from the abdomen

Keep the elbows close to each other

Intermediate

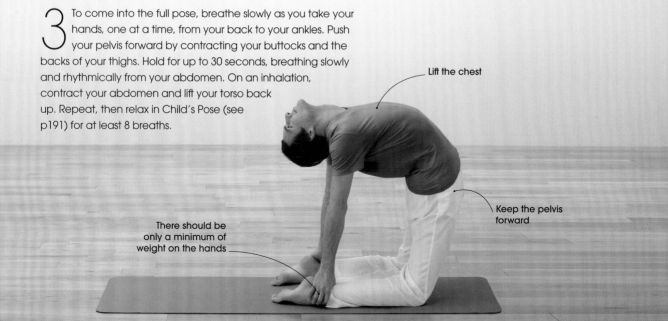

3 To come into the full pose, breathe slowly as you take your hands, one at a time, from your back to your ankles. Push your pelvis forward by contracting your buttocks and the backs of your thighs. Hold for up to 30 seconds, breathing slowly and rhythmically from your abdomen. On an inhalation, contract your abdomen and lift your torso back up. Repeat, then relax in Child's Pose (see p191) for at least 8 breaths.

Lift the chest

Keep the pelvis forward

There should be only a minimum of weight on the hands

Diamond
Intermediate and Advanced

Diamond is a complete backward bend, which you achieve with the help of a strong movement of your arms. It gives a wonderful stretch to the front of the body and revitalizes the area of the solar plexus.

Intermediate

1 Kneel, then sit between your heels, taking your arms behind you. Slowly lower your body onto your elbows, then come into a lying position with your arms behind your head, each hand clasping the opposite elbow. Hold for up to 30 seconds, breathing slowly and rhythmically in your abdomen. Continue with Step 2 or come out of the pose by placing your elbows next to your lower back and pushing yourself up. Then extend your legs in front of you. Relax in Child's Pose (see p191).

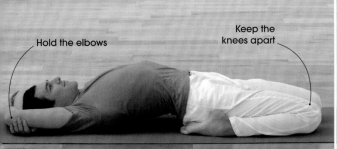

Hold the elbows

Keep the knees apart

Intermediate

2 Place your palms flat on the mat as close to your shoulders as possible. Inhale, push on your arms, and place the top of your head on the floor.

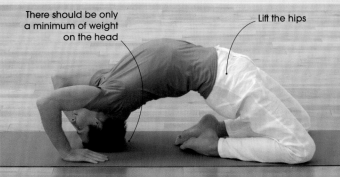

There should be only a minimum of weight on the head

Lift the hips

3 To come into the full pose, with a deep inhalation and another push of your arms, take your head closer to your feet. Move your hands to your feet and push your elbows firmly into the ground. Hold for up to 30 seconds, then release by walking your hands away from your body and lowering your neck to the mat. Repeat, then push yourself up by placing your elbows next to your lower back. Extend your legs in front of you. Relax in Child's Pose (see p191).

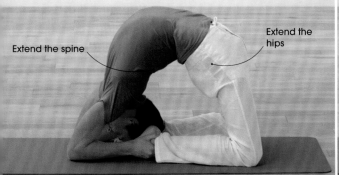

Extend the spine

Extend the hips

Hands On Thighs Advanced Variation

Starting from Diamond Step 2, with an inhalation, slowly lift one arm at a time and place your hands on your thighs so you are balancing on your head and legs. Hold for a few breaths, then release by returning to Diamond Step 2, then lower your neck to the mat. Repeat, then push yourself up by placing your elbows next to your lower back. Extend your legs in front of you. Relax in Child's Pose (see p191).

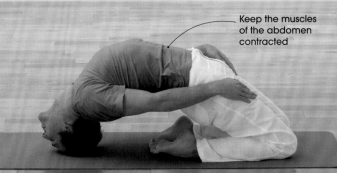

Keep the muscles of the abdomen contracted

Pigeon
All levels

Holding on to your foot by extending your arms over your head in a sitting position is a thrilling experience. It stretches your spine completely and helps to develop an excellent sense of balance.

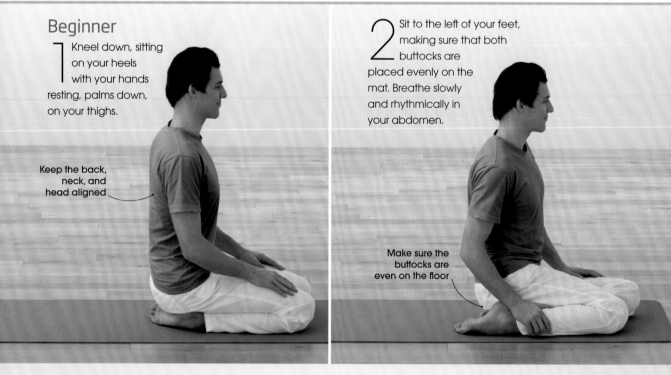

Beginner

1 Kneel down, sitting on your heels with your hands resting, palms down, on your thighs.

Keep the back, neck, and head aligned

2 Sit to the left of your feet, making sure that both buttocks are placed evenly on the mat. Breathe slowly and rhythmically in your abdomen.

Make sure the buttocks are even on the floor

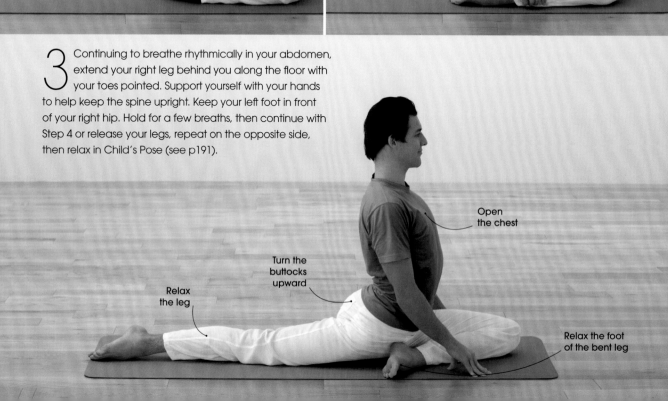

3 Continuing to breathe rhythmically in your abdomen, extend your right leg behind you along the floor with your toes pointed. Support yourself with your hands to help keep the spine upright. Keep your left foot in front of your right hip. Hold for a few breaths, then continue with Step 4 or release your legs, repeat on the opposite side, then relax in Child's Pose (see p191).

Open the chest

Turn the buttocks upward

Relax the leg

Relax the foot of the bent leg

Intermediate

4 Bend your right knee, reach back with your right hand, and then push your right heel against your right buttock. Hold for a few breaths, then continue with Step 5 or repeat on the opposite side, then relax in Child's Pose (see p191).

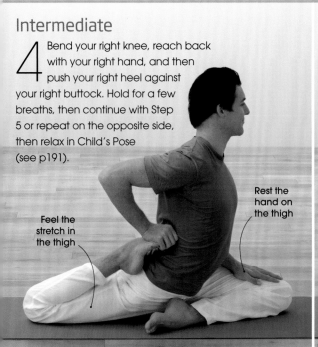

Feel the stretch in the thigh

Rest the hand on the thigh

Advanced

5 Catch the inner edge of your right foot with your right hand. Place your left hand on the floor next to your left hip to help you balance. Keep your breath flowing rhythmically.

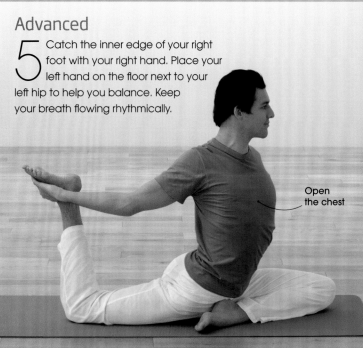

Open the chest

6 Taking your head back, pull your right foot close to your shoulder with your right hand. Continuing to breathe rhythmically, turn your right elbow upward. Stabilize yourself with your left hand on the mat.

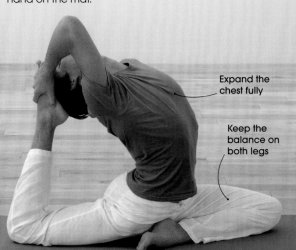

Expand the chest fully

Keep the balance on both legs

7 To come into the full pose, breathe rhythmically to help you balance, bring your left arm over your head, and place your left hand next to your right hand on your right foot. Try to bring your right foot to the top of your head. Hold for a few breaths, then release. Repeat on the opposite side, then relax in Child's Pose (see p191) for 30 seconds.

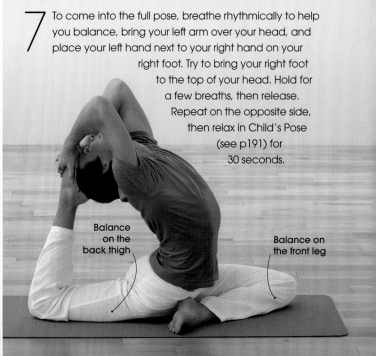

Balance on the back thigh

Balance on the front leg

Crescent Moon
All Levels

One of the main benefits of this asana is the stretch it gives to the hip flexors (iliopsoas) in the pelvis. These are often shortened due to our sedentary life style, and cause stiffness in the lower back.

Beginner

1 Kneel on the floor, then take your right foot forward between your hands. Stretch your left leg back, placing your left knee on the mat. Keep your front calf vertical. Breathe slowly and rhythmically.

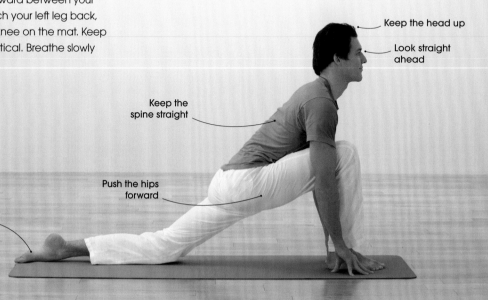

Keep the head up

Look straight ahead

Keep the spine straight

Push the hips forward

Relax the back foot

2 Inhale and take your hands in front of your chest in Prayer Position (see p50). Keep your back vertical and use your bent leg and the toes of your front foot to help you balance. Hold for a few breaths, then continue with Step 3 or release the pose, repeat on the other side, then relax in Child's Pose (see p191).

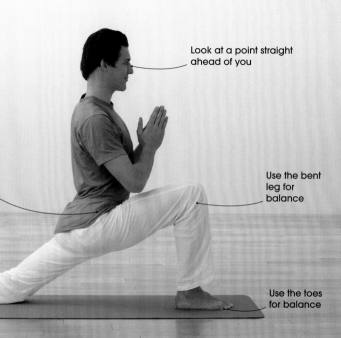

Look at a point straight ahead of you

Push the hips down using the weight of the body

Use the bent leg for balance

Use the toes for balance

Intermediate

3 On an inhalation, take both arms straight up alongside your ears. Hold for up to 30 seconds, breathing slowly and rhythmically. On each inhalation, stretch your arms higher; on each exhalation, try to lower your hips to the floor a little more. Continue with Step 4 or release the pose, repeat on the other side, then relax in Child's Pose (see p191).

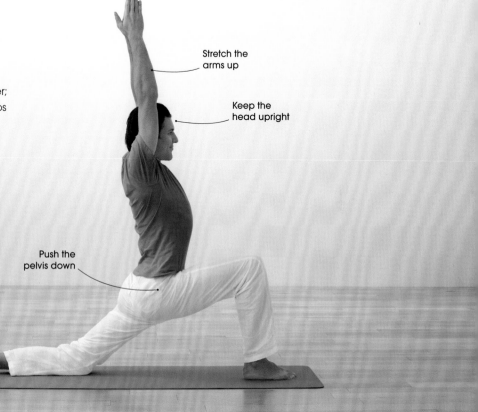

Stretch the arms up

Keep the head upright

Push the pelvis down

Advanced

4 To come into the full pose, on another inhalation, bend backward from your chest. Hold for up to 30 seconds, then repeat on the other side. Relax in Child's Pose (see p191) for at least 8 breaths.

Keep the arms aligned with the ears

Feel the stretch in the back thigh

Push the pelvis forward

Relax the back foot

8 Bow
Dhanurasana

Bow combines the benefits of Cobra (see pp116–118) and Locust (see pp122–123). In this pose, the muscles of the legs and back are activated to form the shape of a bow, while the arms are stretched passively like the string of a bow. Relax afterward in Child's Pose (see p191) for 8 breaths.

Benefits

PHYSICAL

- Tones the muscles of the back.
- Maintains the elasticity of the whole spine.
- Counteracts kyphosis—excessive curvature of the upper back (see p29).
- Strengthens the quadriceps muscles in the front of the thighs.
- Alleviates gastrointestinal disorders.
- Energizes digestion.
- Relieves constipation.
- Energizes the female reproductive system.

MENTAL

- Counteracts mental sluggishness and laziness.

Bow Beginner

1 Lie on your abdomen with both legs and arms stretched out. Bend your right leg and catch hold of your right ankle with your right hand.

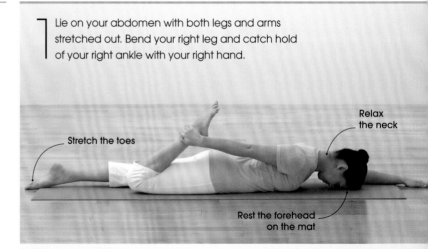

Stretch the toes

Relax the neck

Rest the forehead on the mat

2 With an inhalation, push your right leg up and lift your head. Hold for up to 5 breaths, then release on an exhalation. Repeat with the opposite leg. Relax for a few breaths on your front or in Child's Pose (see p191).

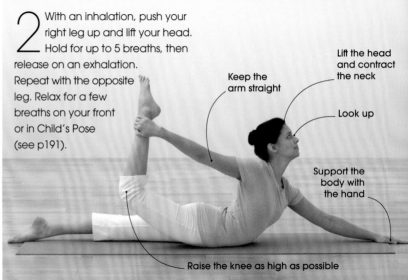

Keep the arm straight

Lift the head and contract the neck

Look up

Support the body with the hand

Raise the knee as high as possible

Bow

Intermediate and Advanced

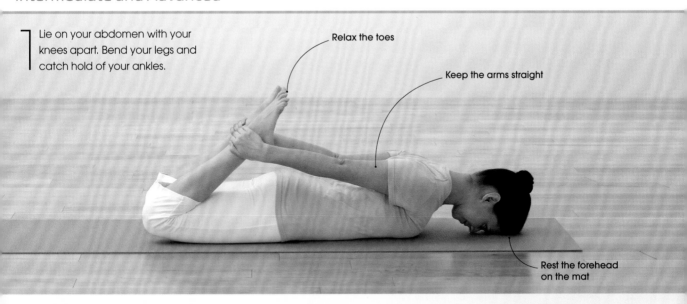

1 Lie on your abdomen with your knees apart. Bend your legs and catch hold of your ankles.

Relax the toes

Keep the arms straight

Rest the forehead on the mat

2 To come into the full pose, on an inhalation, push your feet up until your knees come as high off the mat as possible. Lift your head and contract your neck. Hold for 3–6 breaths, then exhale, release your feet, and lower your knees and forehead back to the mat. Relax in Child's Pose (see p191) for 8 breaths.

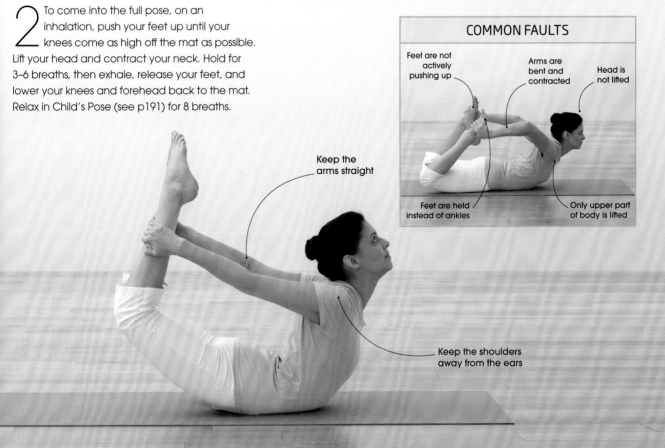

Keep the arms straight

Keep the shoulders away from the ears

COMMON FAULTS

Feet are not actively pushing up

Arms are bent and contracted

Head is not lifted

Feet are held instead of ankles

Only upper part of body is lifted

Bow
Variations

These variations bring complete flexibility to the shoulder joints but require flexible hip and chest muscles. After you have practiced them, stretch back into Child's Pose (see p191) to relax.

Start with

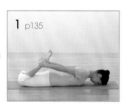

1 p135

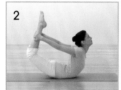

2

Rocking Bow
Intermediate

3 Starting from Bow Step 2, with a strong inhalation, strongly contract your neck and your upper back muscles. Lift your head and chest as high as you can. This creates a backward rocking motion, shifting your weight from your abdomen to your thighs.

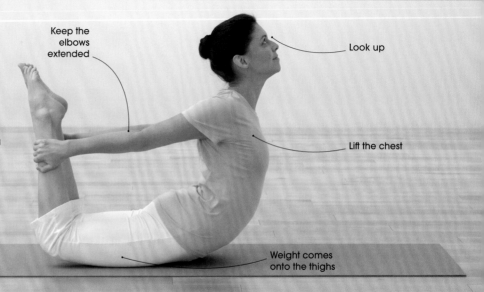

Keep the elbows extended

Look up

Lift the chest

Weight comes onto the thighs

4 With a strong exhalation, use your arms and shoulders to pull your body forward, moving your weight onto your abdomen and chest. Rock forward and back 3–6 times, then exhale, release your feet, and lower your knees and forehead back to the mat. Relax in Child's Pose (see p191) for 30 seconds.

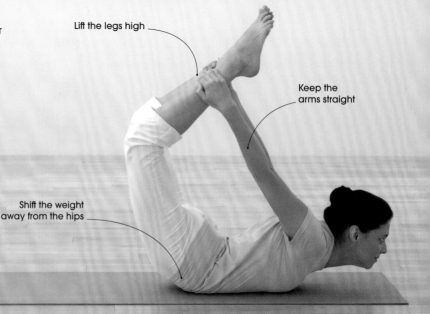

Lift the legs high

Keep the arms straight

Shift the weight away from the hips

One-Handed Bow
Advanced

1 Lie on your abdomen, supporting yourself with your bent left arm. Bend your right leg and catch your right foot just below your big toe with your right hand. Keep your left foot stretched behind you.

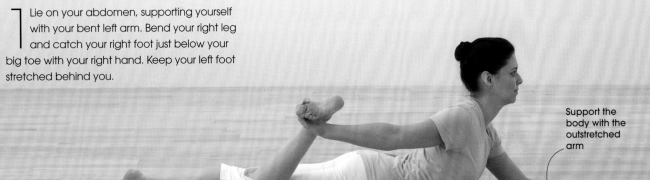

Support the body with the outstretched arm

Stretch the thigh

2 On an inhalation, pull your right foot closer to your shoulder. Straighten your other arm to help push your chest higher into the backward bend.

Lift the head

Look straight ahead

Keep your balance with the outstretched arm

3 Once your foot is close enough to your shoulder, breathe slowly and lift your right elbow, pulling your foot higher up. Hold for a few breaths, then exhale, release your foot, and lower your knee and forehead back to the mat. Repeat on the opposite side, then relax in Child's Pose (see p191).

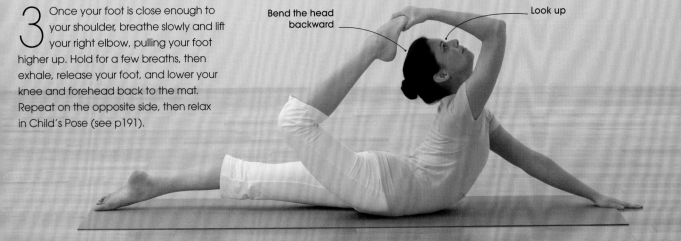

Bend the head backward

Look up

Bow
Variations (continued)

Complete Bow is a truly dynamic pose, to be attempted when you can do One-Handed Bow (see p137). It gives you a powerful anterior stretch, all the way from your throat to your knees.

Complete Bow
Advanced

1 Lying on your abdomen, bend both legs and catch hold of each foot, placing your fingers around your big toes and the tops of your feet. Breathe deeply and slowly.

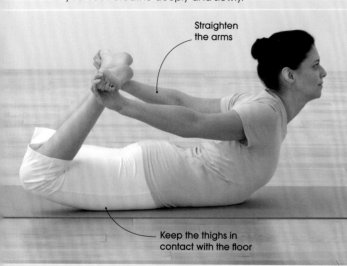

Straighten the arms

Keep the thighs in contact with the floor

2 Rotate your shoulders as you bend your elbows and pull your feet as close to your shoulders as possible. Your thighs will come off the ground. Focus on rhythmical breathing.

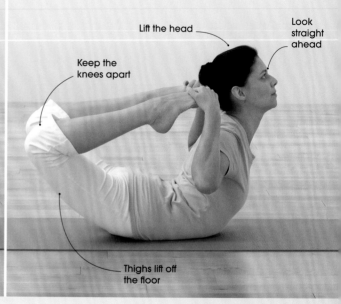

Lift the head

Look straight ahead

Keep the knees apart

Thighs lift off the floor

3 Continue breathing slowly. Once your feet are close enough to your shoulders, lift your elbows forward, in front of your face, pulling your feet even higher. Hold for a few breaths, then exhale, release your feet, and lower your knees and forehead back to the mat. Relax in Child's Pose (see p191).

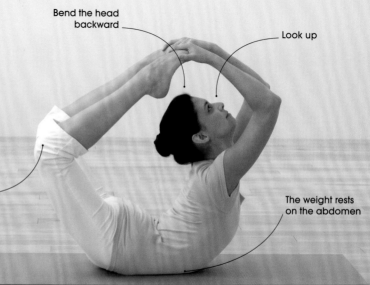

Bend the head backward

Look up

Extend the knees to help lift the feet

The weight rests on the abdomen

Feet to Head
Advanced

Starting from Complete Bow Step 3 (see opposite), breathe slowly and rhythmically as you continue gently pulling your feet until they touch your forehead. Hold for a few breaths, then exhale, release your feet, and lower your knees and forehead back to the mat. Relax in Child's Pose (see p191).

Extend the neck to the maximum

Keep the knees apart

Contract the arms

Feet to Shoulders
Advanced

Starting from Feet to Head (see above), with slow breathing, try to pull your feet gently on top of your shoulders. This requires great flexibility of the spine and shoulders. Hold for a few breaths, then exhale, release your feet, and lower your knees and forehead back to the mat. Relax in Child's Pose (see p191).

Look up

Keep the forearms parallel to the floor

Keep the calves parallel to the floor

Wheel
All Levels

Wheel requires muscle length and muscle strength as well as sense of balance. Being able to hold this pose with deep rhythmical breathing is a sign that you are making good progress in your asanas.

Beginner

1 Lie on your back with your knees bent and your feet a hip-width apart and flat on the mat. Hold your ankles. Breathe deeply and rhythmically.

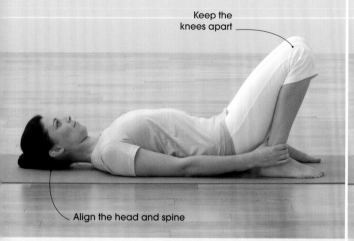

Keep the knees apart

Align the head and spine

2 Keep your head, shoulders, and feet on the floor as you inhale and lift your hips up as high as possible. Hold for a couple of deep, rhythmical breaths, then either continue with Step 3 or lower your hips back to the floor and relax on your back with bent knees (see p189).

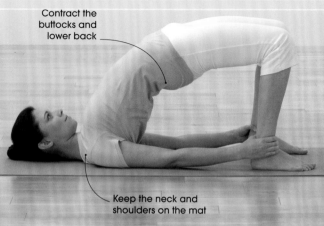

Contract the buttocks and lower back

Keep the neck and shoulders on the mat

Intermediate and Advanced

3 Still breathing deeply and rhythmically, continue lifting your hips and take your hands next to your ears, with your fingers facing your shoulders. Keep your feet parallel to each other.

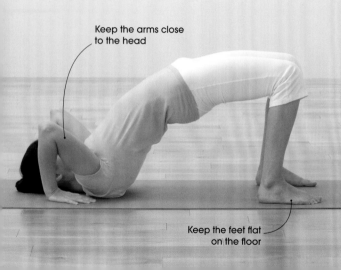

Keep the arms close to the head

Keep the feet flat on the floor

4 Inhale, push on your hands, lift your head, and gently place the top of your head on the floor. Your elbows are pointing backward and your arms bent.

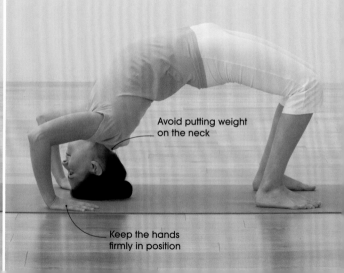

Avoid putting weight on the neck

Keep the hands firmly in position

5 To come into the full pose, on the next inhalation, straighten your arms to lift your torso. If you find it difficult to straighten your arms, try balancing on your toes, then, once your arms are straight, lower your heels. Hold for a few breaths, then come out of the pose by bending your arms and repeating Steps 3, 2, and 1 in that order. Make sure you release the pose before it becomes too tiring, so you have the strength to lower your neck safely back to the floor. Repeat this sequence 1–2 times more, then relax on your back with bent knees (see p189).

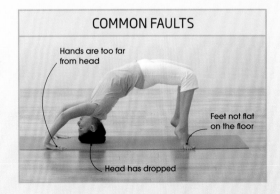

COMMON FAULTS

Hands are too far from head

Feet not flat on the floor

Head has dropped

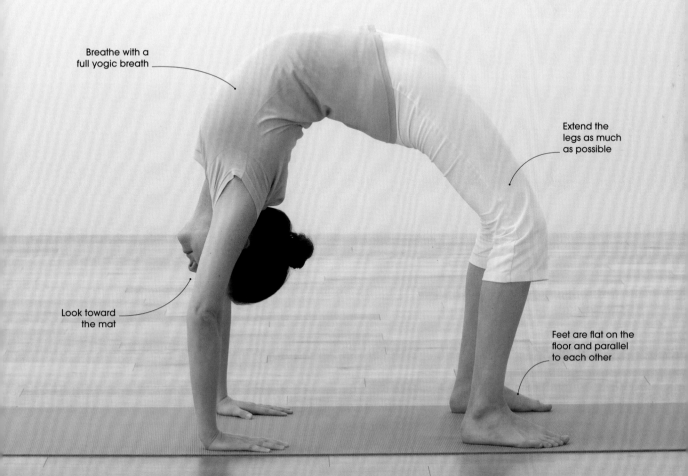

Breathe with a full yogic breath

Extend the legs as much as possible

Look toward the mat

Feet are flat on the floor and parallel to each other

Wheel
Variations

These advanced Wheel variations are best practiced with another person or a teacher standing next to you, ready to hold your hips in case you start falling to one side.

Start with

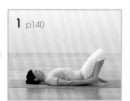 **1** p140

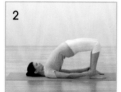 **2**

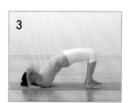 **3**

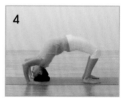 **4**

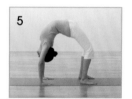 **5**

One Leg Up Advanced

Starting from Wheel Step 5, shift your weight to your right leg. On an inhalation, lift your left leg. Hold your breath, then lower the leg back to the floor on an exhalation. Repeat on the opposite side, then either continue with One Arm Up (see right) or come out of the pose by bending your arms and repeating Wheel Steps 3, 2, and 1 in that order. Relax on your back with bent knees (see p189).

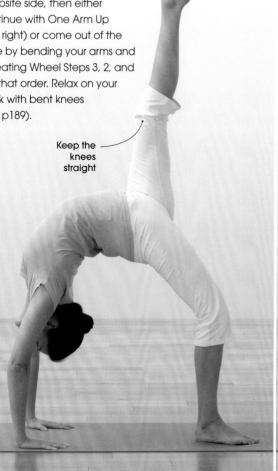

Stretch the toes

Keep the knees straight

One Arm Up Advanced

Starting from Wheel Step 5, shift your weight to your left arm. Inhale and lift your right arm, then place your right hand on your right thigh, fingers turned inward. Hold your breath for a few seconds; then, on an exhalation, lower your right arm back to the floor. Repeat on the opposite side, then come out of the pose by bending your arms and repeating Wheel Steps 3, 2, and 1 in that order. Relax on your back with bent knees (see p189).

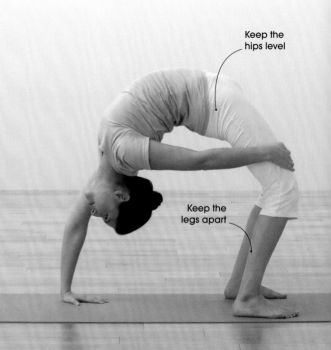

Keep the hips level

Keep the legs apart

Full Wheel from Standing
Advanced

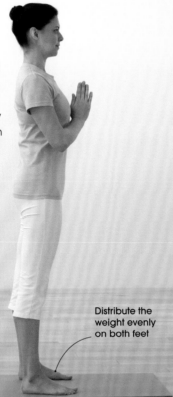

1 Stand near the front of the mat with your legs 20 in (50 cm) apart and your feet turned slightly outward. Hold your hands in Prayer Position (see p50) in front of your chest.

Distribute the weight evenly on both feet

2 Inhale and lift your arms over your head. Drop your head back and start bending backward, holding your arms out straight behind you.

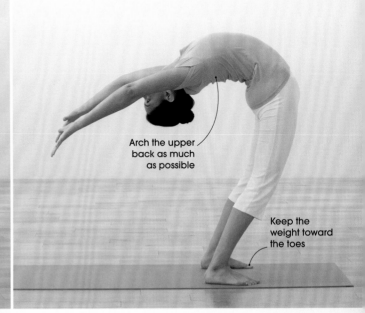

Arch the upper back as much as possible

Keep the weight toward the toes

3 Bend your knees slightly and continue bending backward, taking your extended arms closer to the floor. Hold your breath and keep your balance by shifting your body weight as far forward as possible.

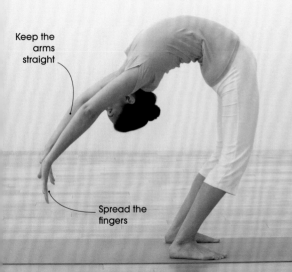

Keep the arms straight

Spread the fingers

4 Once you are near the floor, let your body weight shift gently toward your arms. As soon as your hands meet the floor, bend your elbows slightly to protect your wrists. Take a few breaths, then return to Step 1 by inhaling and quickly shifting your weight to the front. Alternatively, bend your elbows and come up by following Wheel Steps 3, 2, and 1, in that order. Relax on your back with bent knees (see p189).

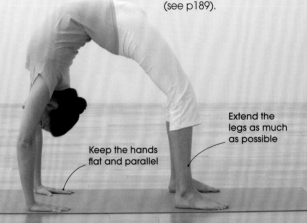

Extend the legs as much as possible

Keep the hands flat and parallel

9 Half Spinal Twist
Ardha Matsyendrasana

Lateral rotation is important for achieving complete flexibility of the spine. These twisting asanas work on the rotation of all the vertebrae, as well as the hip joint. Follow each of them with Child's Pose (see p191) as a relaxing counterpose. This asana is named after the great yogic sage, Matsyendranath.

Benefits

PHYSICAL

• Helps to improve the flexibility of the spine.

• Helps to tone the roots of the spinal nerves.

• Helps to energize the gastrointestinal system.

• Enhances the functioning of the large intestine.

• Improves the appetite.

MENTAL

• Rotation or twisting of the spine is not a common movement in daily life. By exploring this unusual movement, your mind will also become more flexible and adaptable.

Half Spinal Twist Beginner

1 Sit with your legs extended straight in front of you and take both arms behind your back. Place your hands palms down, with your fingers pointing backward. Breathe rhythmically in the abdomen.

Open the chest

Relax the shoulders

Keep the feet straight yet relaxed

Keep the arms straight

2 Place your left foot flat on the mat outside your right calf. Inhale and lift your right arm straight up.

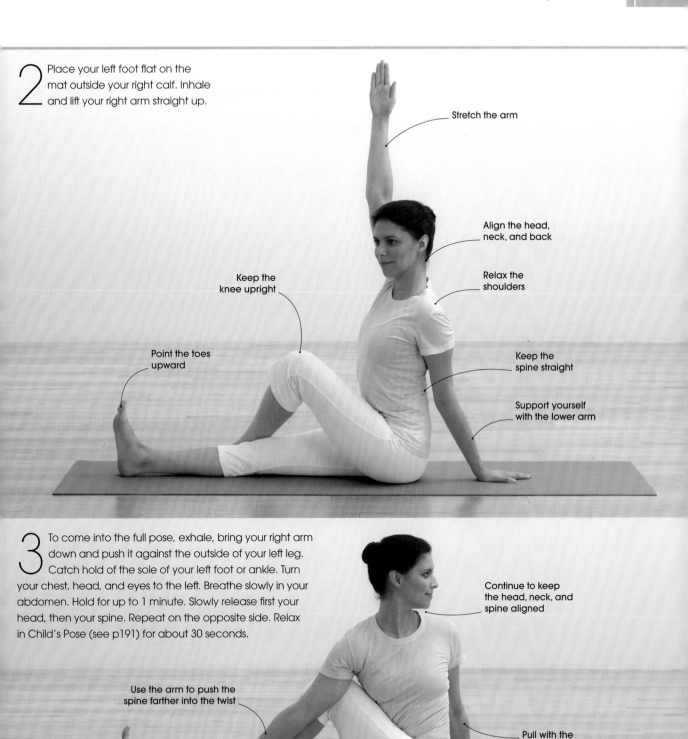

Stretch the arm

Align the head, neck, and back

Keep the knee upright

Relax the shoulders

Point the toes upward

Keep the spine straight

Support yourself with the lower arm

3 To come into the full pose, exhale, bring your right arm down and push it against the outside of your left leg. Catch hold of the sole of your left foot or ankle. Turn your chest, head, and eyes to the left. Breathe slowly in your abdomen. Hold for up to 1 minute. Slowly release first your head, then your spine. Repeat on the opposite side. Relax in Child's Pose (see p191) for about 30 seconds.

Continue to keep the head, neck, and spine aligned

Use the arm to push the spine farther into the twist

Pull with the arm to allow the chest to turn farther

Half Spinal Twist
Intermediate and Advanced

The lumbar area does not twist easily, so you need to rotate the cervical and thoracic areas of your spine. Keeping your chest open and your neck straight is the best basis for a good twist.

1 Start by sitting on your heels and placing your palms face down on your thighs.

2 Still with your palms on your thighs, adjust yourself so you are sitting to the right of your feet, with your buttocks even on the floor.

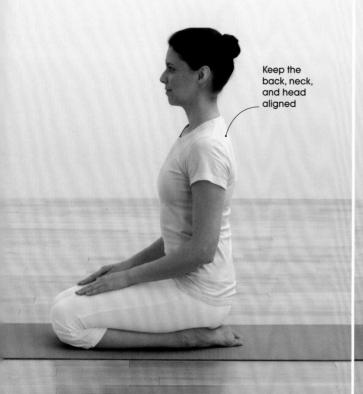

Keep the back, neck, and head aligned

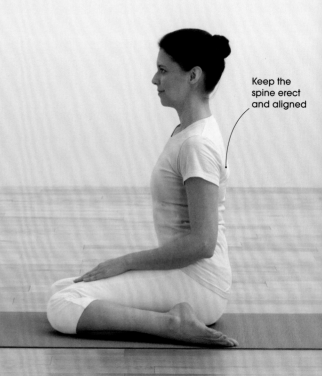

Keep the spine erect and aligned

3 Take your left foot over your right thigh, placing it flat on the mat close to your knee. Support your body with your left arm behind your back. Inhale and lift your right arm straight up.

4 To come into the full pose, exhale, bring your right arm down, and push it against the outside of your left knee as you try to catch hold of the sole of your left foot or ankle. Turn your chest, head, and eyes to the left. Breathe slowly in your abdomen. Hold the pose for up to 1 minute. Slowly release first your head, then your spine. Repeat on the opposite side, then either practice the variations (see pp148–149) or relax in Child's Pose (see p191) for about 30 seconds.

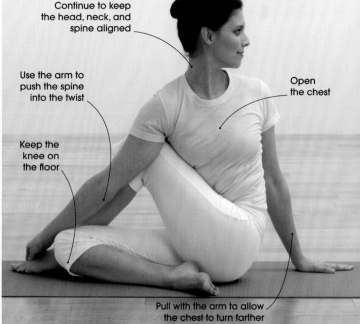

COMMON FAULTS

Outstretched arm does not reach either the ankle or the foot

Chin is too high

Knee is not on the floor

Supporting arm is too far forward

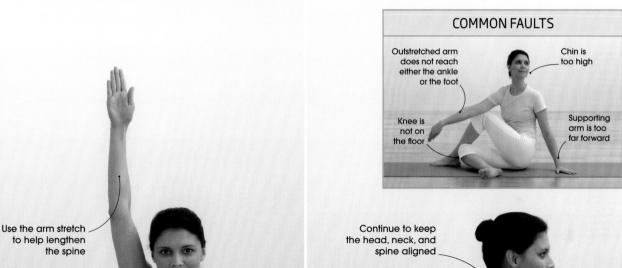

Use the arm stretch to help lengthen the spine

Keep the buttock on the mat

Continue to keep the head, neck, and spine aligned

Use the arm to push the spine into the twist

Keep the knee on the floor

Open the chest

Pull with the arm to allow the chest to turn farther

Half Spinal Twist
Variations

These variations increase both the rotation of the spine and the stretch in the abductor muscles on the outside of your thighs. Only practice them if you can keep your back, neck, and head upright.

Start with

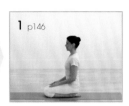

1 p146

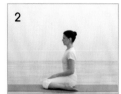

2

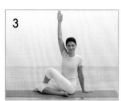

3

Wrist Grasp
Advanced

Starting from Intermediate Half Spinal Twist Step 3, take your right arm through the space between your left knee and your right leg. Hold your left hand or wrist. Hold with slow abdominal breathing for up to 2 minutes. Repeat on the opposite side. Relax in Child's Pose (see p191).

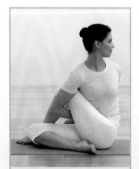

Front view This view shows clearly the full opening of the chest in the pose.

Ankle Clasp Advanced

Starting from Wrist Grasp (see left), take your left foot closer to your hip. Place your left arm against your back, and try to hold your left ankle. Hold your right knee with your right hand and use your right arm as a lever to help you to twist to the left. Breathe slowly and hold for up to 2 minutes. Repeat on the opposite side. Relax in Child's Pose (see p191).

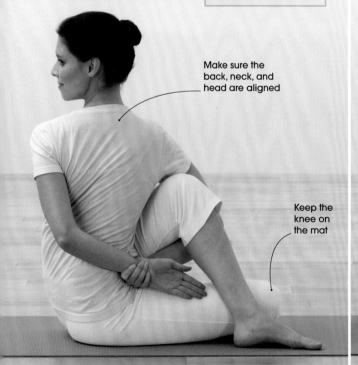

Make sure the back, neck, and head are aligned

Keep the knee on the mat

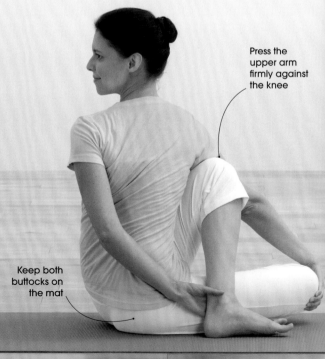

Press the upper arm firmly against the knee

Keep both buttocks on the mat

Start with

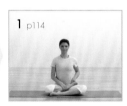

1 p114

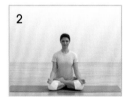

2

Full Spinal Twist Advanced

This is Purna Matsyendrasana or Full Spinal
Twist. Starting from Lotus Step 2, lift your left leg
and catch hold of your left foot with your right
hand. Keep your left arm behind your back.
Turn your head to the left and look over your
left shoulder. Hold for up to 1 minute with
rhythmical breathing. Slowly release first your
head, then your spine. Repeat on the opposite
side, then relax in Child's Pose (see p191).

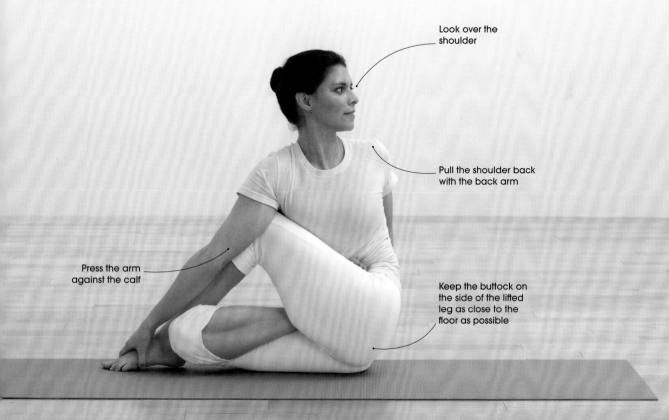

Look over the
shoulder

Pull the shoulder back
with the back arm

Press the arm
against the calf

Keep the buttock on
the side of the lifted
leg as close to the
floor as possible

10a Crow
Kakasana

Strengthening the arms and the shoulder girdle is a main concern in any exercise program. Instead of using weights, the Yogis developed balancing asanas such as Crow and its variations. In these, the body weight shifts from the lower body to the upper body. Relax afterward in Child's Pose (see p191).

Benefits

PHYSICAL

- Helps to develop strength and flexibility in the wrists.
- Strengthens the tricep muscles.
- Strengthens the shoulder muscles.
- The variations further strengthen the muscles of the legs, hips, and back.

MENTAL

- When you are practicing this pose, you have to evaluate how much of your body weight you can place on your arms and hands. If you place too little weight on them, you will not be able to lift your feet off the floor. After a period of testing and hesitation, one concentrated, determined movement will lift you into the pose. Crow therefore helps to develop your determination as well as your powers of concentration.

Crow Beginner

1 Sit in a squatting position with your legs and feet apart. Taking your shoulders in front of your knees, place your palms on the mat in front of you. Keep your arms slightly bent and adopt the correct position for your hands and elbows (see right). Breathe slowly and rhythmically.

Hand and Elbow Position
Spread your fingers wide apart, turn your wrists inward, and bend your elbows outward.

Knees are wide apart

Look straight ahead

2 Come up onto your toes, lifting your hips, and keeping your knees pressed firmly against your upper arms. Continue breathing rhythmically in the abdomen.

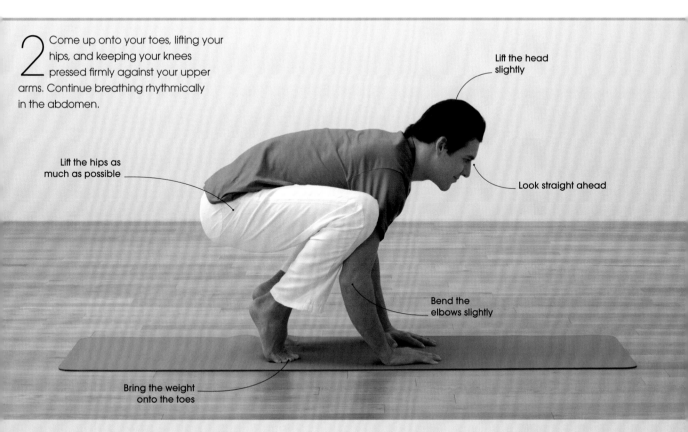

Lift the head slightly

Look straight ahead

Lift the hips as much as possible

Bend the elbows slightly

Bring the weight onto the toes

3 Breathing more deeply, focus on a point in front of you, then slowly move forward, shifting your weight away from your feet and onto your wrists. Your elbows are slightly bent and your knees are resting on your upper arms. Continue with Step 4 (see p152) or hold for a few moments, then exhale and return to a squatting position. Relax in Child's Pose (see p191).

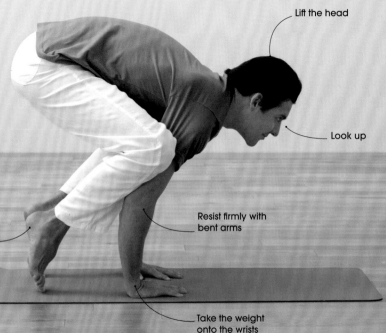

Lift the head

Look up

Resist firmly with bent arms

Take most of the weight off the feet

Take the weight onto the wrists

Crow
Intermediate and Advanced

The Crow variation (see right) is far simpler to perform than it looks. What you need is a very steady base to support the weight of your legs. Side Crow also helps to develop lateral balancing.

Start with

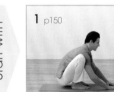

1 p150

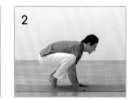

2

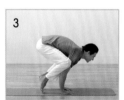

3

4 If your wrists are strong enough, come into the full pose. Starting from Crow Step 3, inhale, hold your breath, then slowly move your weight farther forward until your feet lift off the floor. Balance for a few moments, then exhale, and return to Step 2. Once you can achieve the full pose, hold it as you breathe rhythmically for up to 30 seconds, then relax in Child's Pose (see p191).

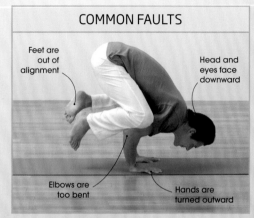

COMMON FAULTS

Feet are out of alignment

Head and eyes face downward

Elbows are too bent

Hands are turned outward

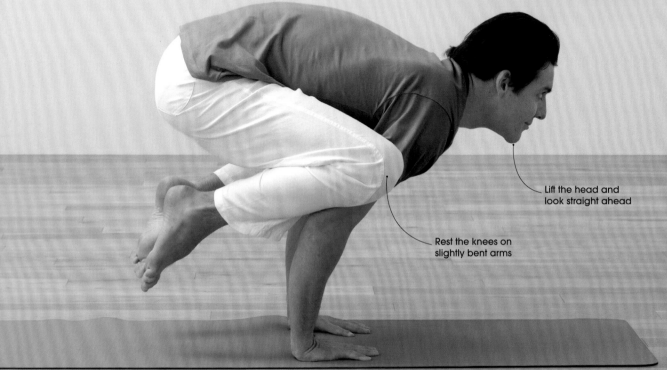

Lift the head and look straight ahead

Rest the knees on slightly bent arms

Side Crow Advanced Variation

1 Starting from a kneeling squat, place both hands flat on the floor, 20 in (50 cm) apart, to the right of your legs. Walk both feet to the left.

2 Make sure your feet are 20 in (50 cm) from your left hand and in line with your hands. Bend your knees and take your legs onto the top of your left elbow. Inhale and hold your breath as you shift your weight forward until your feet come off the floor.

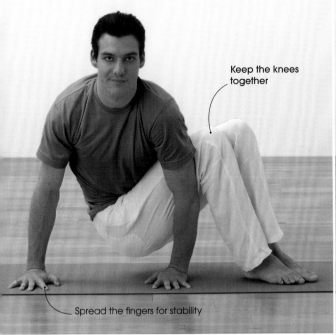

Keep the knees together

Spread the fingers for stability

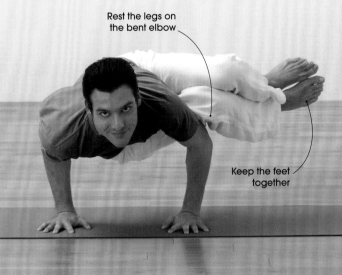

Rest the legs on the bent elbow

Keep the feet together

3 Breathing deeply and rhythmically, shift the weight of your head, torso, feet, and legs forward as you slowly extend your legs. Hold for as long as deep rhythmical breathing allows you, then bend your knees and come back to a kneeling squat. Repeat on the other side, then relax in Child's Pose (see p191).

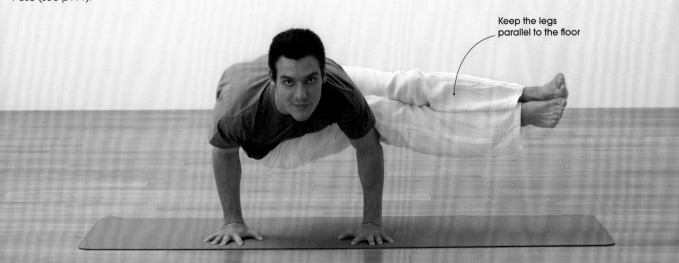

Keep the legs parallel to the floor

10b Peacock
Mayurasana

In this pose, your body resembles a peacock with its feathers spread out behind. It is an excellent balancing exercise. In addition, you will have strengthened many of the muscles in your body and will have toned your lungs and abdominal organs. Relax afterward in Child's Pose (see p191).

Benefits

PHYSICAL

• Strengthens the muscles of the legs, arms, back, abdomen, shoulders, and neck.

• Tones the lungs.

• Tones the abdominal organs.

• Helps to overcome constipation.

• Gives the whole body a powerful tonic.

MENTAL

• The strong muscular effort, deep breathing, and keen concentration required for this pose help to overcome sluggishness (tamas, see p212) as well as hyperactivity (rajas, see p212).

Peacock Beginner

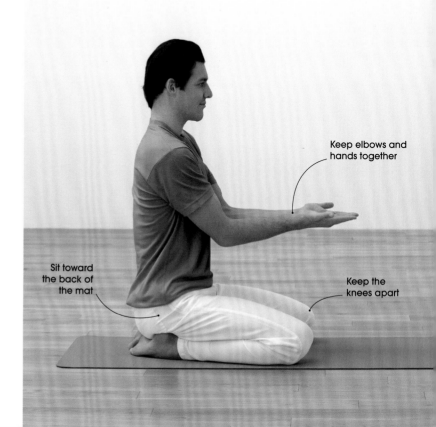

1 Kneel down with your knees wide apart, then sit between your heels. Hold your arms in front of you, elbows bent, keeping your elbows and hands together. Breathe deeply and rhythmically.

Keep elbows and hands together

Sit toward the back of the mat

Keep the knees apart

2 Lean forward, lifting your hips and placing your palms on the mat close to your knees, fingers pointing backward. Keeping your elbows together, place your upper abdomen against them. For some women this may be difficult, in which case, keep your elbows farther apart.

3 Slowly lean forward and lower your forehead to the floor. Keep your abdomen pressed tightly against your elbows and continue breathing rhythmically.

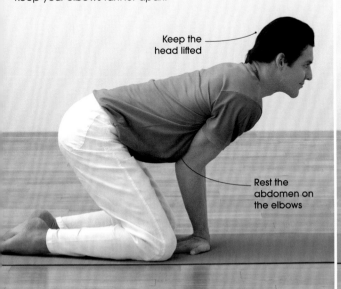

Keep the head lifted

Rest the abdomen on the elbows

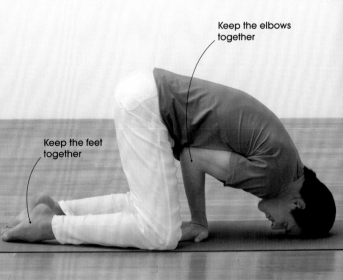

Keep the elbows together

Keep the feet together

4 Stretch one leg out, and then the other. Tuck your toes under. Resist the pressure of your elbows with your abdominal muscles. Continue with Step 5 (see p156) or come down by exhaling, then lowering your feet and knees to the floor. Sit up and shake out your wrists, then relax in Child's Pose (see p191).

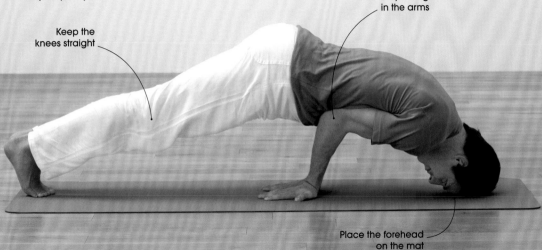

Keep the knees straight

Stay strong in the arms

Place the forehead on the mat

Peacock
Intermediate and Advanced

Each asana acts on specific pressure points of the body, allowing the release of pent-up prana, or vital energy (see pp178-179). Peacock helps prana to circulate from the solar plexus throughout the whole body.

Start with

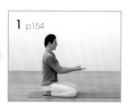

1 p154

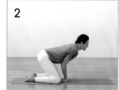

2

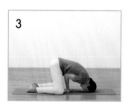

3

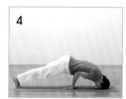

4

Intermediate

5 Starting from Peacock Step 4, on an inhalation, lift your head and chest. Take one more deep breath and prepare to contract the muscles of your legs, back, abdomen, and neck. Continue with Step 6 or come down by exhaling and lowering your feet and knees to the floor. Sit up and shake out your wrists, then relax in Child's Pose (see p191).

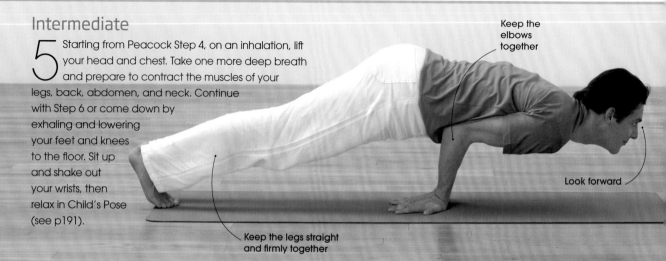

Keep the elbows together

Look forward

Keep the legs straight and firmly together

Advanced

6 To come into the final pose, after the deepest possible inhalation, hold your breath, make your body stiff, and tiptoe forward until your legs come off the floor. Exhale, then lower your feet and knees to the floor. Sit up and shake out your wrists, then relax in Child's Pose (see p191).

COMMON FAULTS

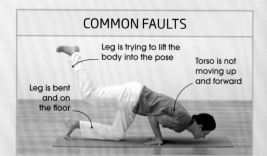

Leg is trying to lift the body into the pose

Torso is not moving up and forward

Leg is bent and on the floor

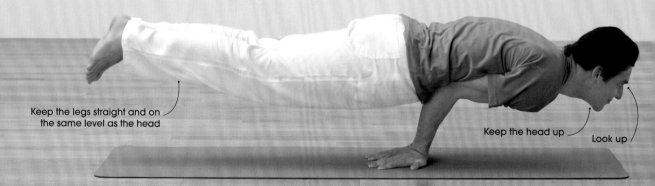

Keep the legs straight and on the same level as the head

Keep the head up

Look up

Head to Floor Advanced Variation

Starting from Peacock Step 6, continue shifting your weight forward until your forehead touches the mat and your legs come high off the floor. Try to hold for 3 breaths, then release. Exhale, then lower your feet and knees to the floor. Sit up and shake out your wrists. Relax in Child's Pose (see p191).

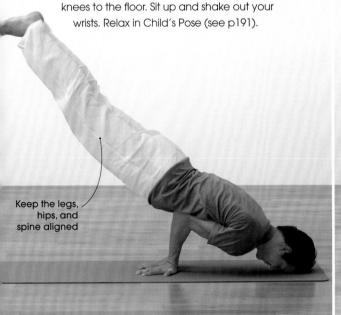

Keep the legs, hips, and spine aligned

2 Move your body forward until you are balancing on your knees. Place your palms flat, with your fingers pointing toward your legs.

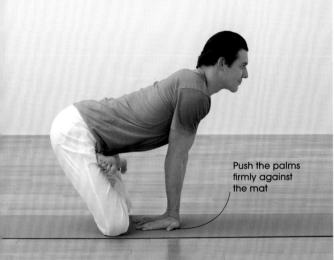

Push the palms firmly against the mat

Lotus Peacock Advanced Variation

1 Sit cross-legged; come into Lotus (see p114) by lifting your left foot onto the top of your right thigh, then your right foot onto the top of your left thigh.

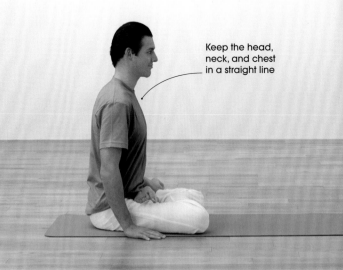

Keep the head, neck, and chest in a straight line

3 Bend your elbows and place them against your abdomen. Inhale and move your body forward, lifting your head and chest together with your bent legs. Hold for up to 3 breaths, then come down by following Steps 2 and 1 in that order. Repeat with your legs crossed the other way. Relax in Child's Pose (see p191).

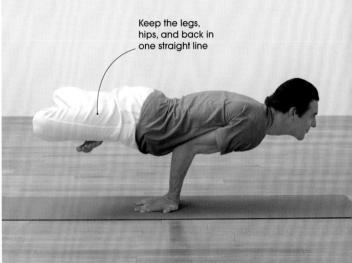

Keep the legs, hips, and back in one straight line

Standing Balances
All Levels

Standing on one leg demands concentration and single-mindedness rather than physical prowess. To help you find your point of balance, alternate your weight between your heel and toes.

Tree Beginner

1 Stand up straight, focusing on a spot in front of you for balance. Breathe slowly from your abdomen. Lift your left foot and place it against your right thigh. Point your left knee outward.

2 When you feel secure in your balance, release the hold on your foot and place your hands in Prayer Position (see p50) in front of your chest. Keep up the rhythmical breathing.

3 With an inhalation, slowly lift your arms. Hold the pose for up to 1 minute. Release, then repeat on the opposite side. Practice another standing asana (see pp159–169) or go directly to final relaxation (see pp192–193).

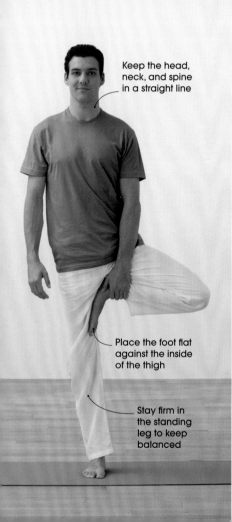

Keep the head, neck, and spine in a straight line

Place the foot flat against the inside of the thigh

Stay firm in the standing leg to keep balanced

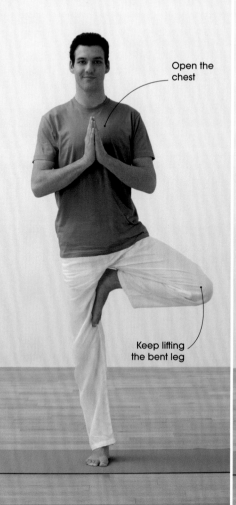

Open the chest

Keep lifting the bent leg

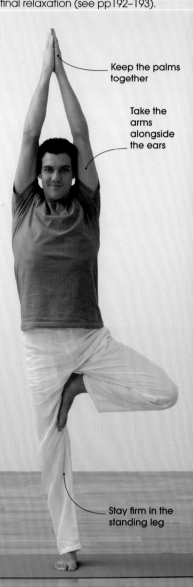

Keep the palms together

Take the arms alongside the ears

Stay firm in the standing leg

Half Lotus Tree
Intermediate Variation

1 Stand up straight, focusing on a spot in front of you to help you keep your balance. Lift your left foot and place it on top of your right thigh in Half Lotus. Release your hold on your foot and take your arms alongside your body. Press firmly into the foot of the standing leg.

2 Slowly lift your arms. Hold for up to 1 minute, breathing rhythmically, then release and repeat on the opposite side. Practice another standing asana (see pp159–169) or go directly to final relaxation (see pp192–193).

Eagle Intermediate

Stand with both knees slightly bent. Place your right knee on top of your left knee and lock your left foot behind your right calf. Place your left upper arm inside your right elbow and bring your palms together in front of your face. Hold for up to 30 seconds, breathing rhythmically. Release and repeat on the opposite side. Practice another standing asana (see pp160–169) or go directly to final relaxation (see pp192–193).

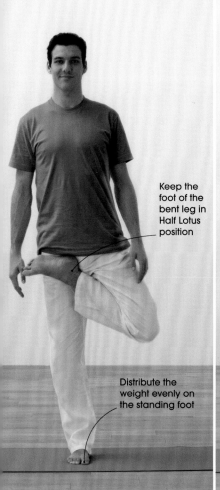

Keep the foot of the bent leg in Half Lotus position

Distribute the weight evenly on the standing foot

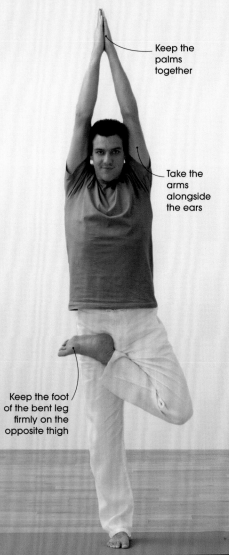

Keep the palms together

Take the arms alongside the ears

Keep the foot of the bent leg firmly on the opposite thigh

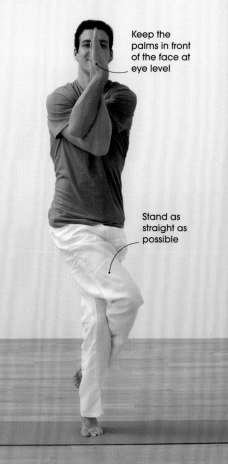

Keep the palms in front of the face at eye level

Stand as straight as possible

Dancing Lord Siva
All Levels

Focusing on the vertical position of the leg and arm on one side of the body creates a stable base. Then you can easily develop the backward bending movement on the other side of the body.

Beginner and Intermediate

1 Stand firmly on both feet. Balance on your left foot, lift your right ankle, and grasp it with your right hand. Establish your balance by breathing slowly and rhythmically.

2 With an inhalation, stretch your left arm up, taking it alongside your left ear. Extend your elbow and stretch your fingers upward. Look firmly at a point in front of you, breathe slowly and rhythmically, and affirm your balance on your left foot.

3 Push your right foot backward as you lean slightly forward with your upper body. Breathe deeply and rhythmically. Hold for up to 30 seconds, then release and repeat on the opposite side. Continue with Step 4, or practice Standing Forward Bend (see pp162–163) or Triangle (see pp164–169), or go directly to final relaxation (see pp192–193).

Concentrate on a spot in front of you

Keep both thighs parallel to each other

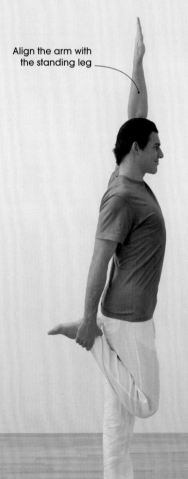

Align the arm with the standing leg

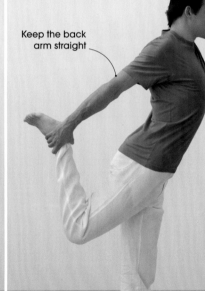

Keep the arm vertical and alongside the ear

Keep the back arm straight

Keep the weight firmly on the standing foot

Advanced

4 Starting from Dancing Lord Siva Step 3, pull your right foot close to your right shoulder until you can lift your elbow. Rotate your wrist so you are holding the upper part of your foot. Breathe deeply and rhythmically. Hold for up to 30 seconds, then release and repeat on the opposite side.

5 To come into the full pose, bring your left arm over your head and lower your left hand to place it on your right foot so that you are holding your foot with both hands. Hold the pose for up to 30 seconds, breathing deeply and rhythmically, then release and repeat on the opposite side. Practice Standing Forward Bend (see pp162–163) or Triangle (see pp164–169), or go directly to final relaxation (see pp192–193).

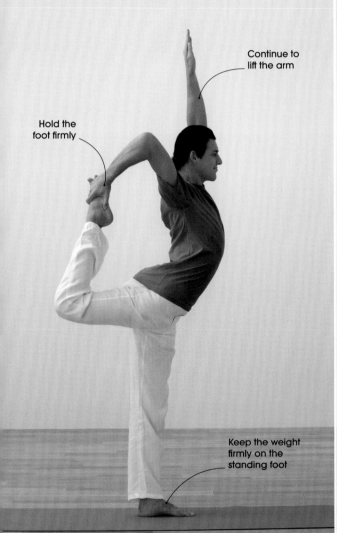

Continue to lift the arm

Hold the foot firmly

Keep the weight firmly on the standing foot

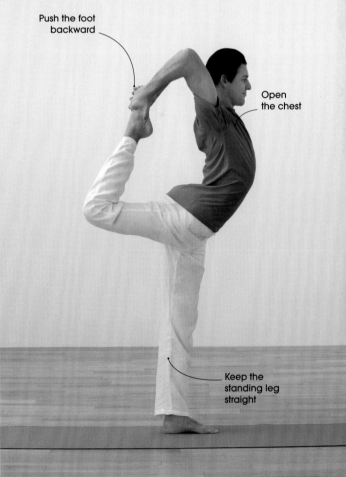

Push the foot backward

Open the chest

Keep the standing leg straight

11 Standing Forward Bend
Pada Hasthasana

If you notice that your legs are stiff from too much sitting, practise this Standing Forward Bend. Using the pull of gravity, this pose lengthens the muscles and ligaments of the entire posterior of your body—from heels to the middle of the back. It also prepares you for Triangle (see pp164–169).

Benefits

PHYSICAL

- Lengthens the muscles in the legs, hips, and lower back.
- Moderately increases the blood supply to the brain.
- Progressively trims the waist when accompanied by proper diet.
- Helps to overcome constipation.

MENTAL

- The stimulation of the spine, the activated sense of balance, and the extra blood supply to the brain produced by this pose all bring relief from tamas (see p212), a state of low energy characterized by sluggishness, inertia, sleepiness, forgetfulness, and depression.

CAUTION If the backs of your knees are over-extended, you should focus on keeping your knees straight without pushing them backward.

Standing Forward Bend All Levels

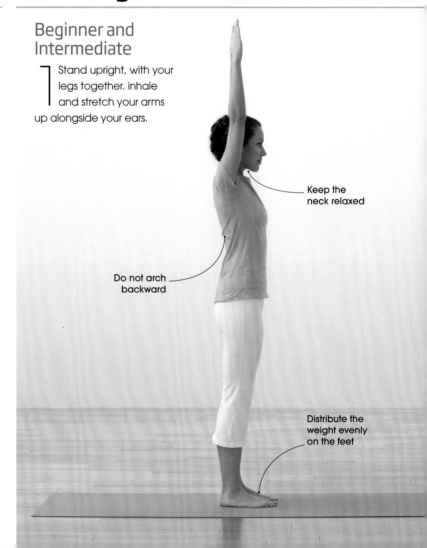

Beginner and Intermediate

1 Stand upright, with your legs together. inhale and stretch your arms up alongside your ears.

Keep the neck relaxed

Do not arch backward

Distribute the weight evenly on the feet

2 Exhale and bend forward from the hips so that you make a horizontal line with your arms and upper body.

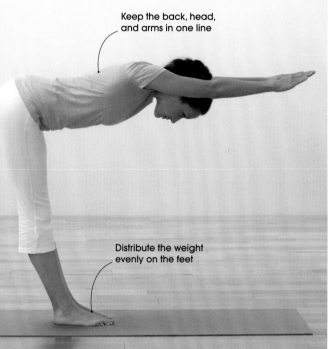

Keep the back, head, and arms in one line

Distribute the weight evenly on the feet

3 Continue exhaling and bending forward. Catch hold of your ankles or calves, or hold onto your big toes in the Classical Foothold (see below). Hold for up to 1 minute with slow rhythmical breathing, then either continue with Step 4 or inhale and come back up, with your arms and head hanging, then return to standing. Follow this with Triangle (see pp164–169).

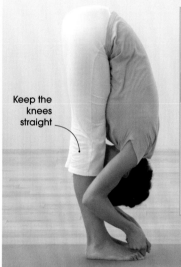

Keep the knees straight

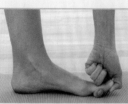

Classical Foothold
Wrap the index finger around the big toe and place the thumb underneath it. Curl the remaining three fingers against the palm.

Advanced

4 If you can hold your toes, come into the full pose by bringing your arms behind your knees and holding your elbows. On an exhalation, push your arms down along your calves. Alternatively, for a greater stretch in the legs, slide the palms of your hands under your feet (see below). Hold either position for up to 1 minute with slow rhythmical breathing, then come back up, with your arms and head hanging, then return to standing. Follow this with Triangle (see pp164–169).

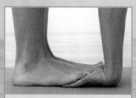

Alternative Foothold
Slide the palms under the feet.

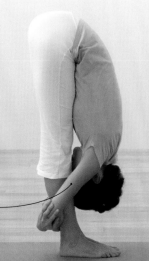

Increase the stretch in the spine by pushing the arms farther down

COMMON FAULTS

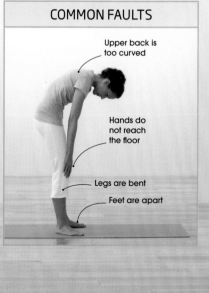

Upper back is too curved

Hands do not reach the floor

Legs are bent

Feet are apart

12 Triangle
Trikonasana

Triangle's lateral bend stretches and strengthens several muscles on the side of the body at the same time. It also helps with balance. It is the last of the twelve basic asanas in the cycle. After you have practised Triangle, end your session with final relaxation (see pp192-193) in order to reap all the benefits of your practice.

Benefits

PHYSICAL

• Increases the sideways mobility of the lumbar and thoracic areas of the spine.

• Strengthens and lengthens the muscles of the legs and back.

• Tones the spinal nerves.

• Tones the abdominal organs.

• Improves the movement of food through the intestines and so invigorates the appetite.

MENTAL

• Working the muscles of the legs and back while still breathing calmly in the abdomen and consciously trying to relax presents both a physical and a mental challenge. Triangle can teach you how to face a challenging task while staying mentally calm and detached.

• Strengthens concentration and mental determination.

Triangle All Levels

Beginner

1 Stand with your legs twice shoulder-width apart. Turn your left foot to the left and then align it with the instep of your right foot. Breathe deeply and slowly.

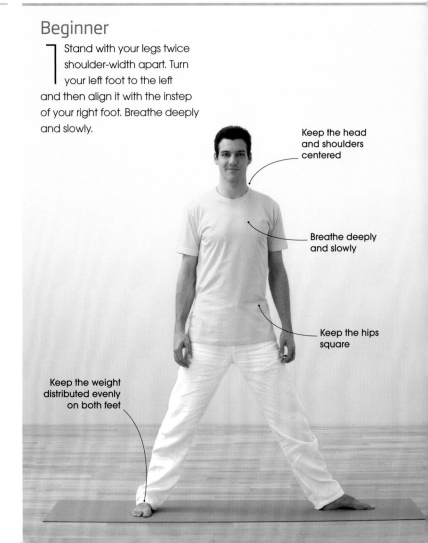

Keep the head and shoulders centered

Breathe deeply and slowly

Keep the hips square

Keep the weight distributed evenly on both feet

2 Inhale and take your right arm up alongside your right ear.

Focus on the stretch from the foot to the raised hand

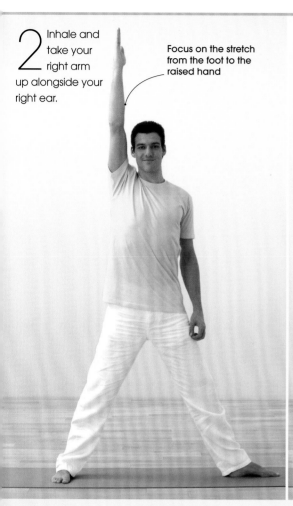

3 If you are unable to reach over your head without bending your leg (see intermediate Step 3), exhale and bend your trunk to the left. Bend your left leg, and place your left hand on your left foot. Hold for up to 1 minute, then repeat on the opposite side. Follow with final relaxation (see pp192–193).

Align the hips, trunk, and arm in one horizontal line

Look up

Turn the face forward

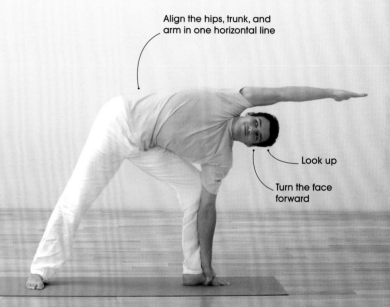

Intermediate and Advanced

3 If you are able to reach over your head without bending your leg, come into the full pose from Step 2. Exhale and bend to the left, keeping your left knee straight. Catch hold of your ankle or calf. Hold for up to 1 minute, then repeat on the opposite side. Follow with final relaxation (see pp192–193).

Do not lean on the lower hand

Keep some weight on the back foot

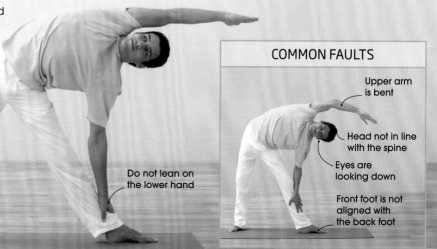

COMMON FAULTS

Upper arm is bent

Head not in line with the spine

Eyes are looking down

Front foot is not aligned with the back foot

Triangle
Variations

These variations add first a hip rotation and then a spinal twist to the lateral bend that you do when you practice Triangle. This combination of movements gives your back a complete workout.

Simple Hip Twist Beginner

1 Stand with your legs about twice shoulder-width apart. Turn your left foot to the left and your right foot slightly inward. Interlock your fingers behind your back. Inhale deeply.

2 With an exhalation, bend your body over your left leg, bringing your forehead to your left knee. Breathe rhythmically, holding for up to 1 minute, then repeat on the opposite side. Follow with final relaxation (see pp192–193).

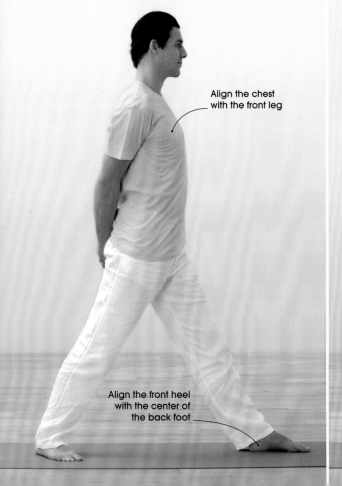

Align the chest with the front leg

Align the front heel with the center of the back foot

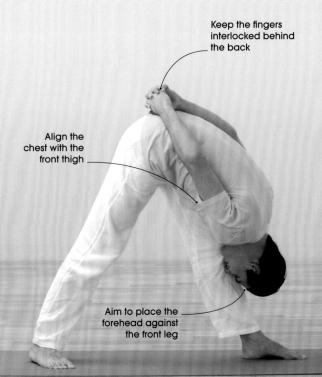

Keep the fingers interlocked behind the back

Align the chest with the front thigh

Aim to place the forehead against the front leg

Triangle with Spinal Twist
Intermediate

1 Stand with your legs about twice shoulder-width apart. Turn your right foot to the right and your left foot slightly inward. Lift your arms parallel to the floor and twist your body as far as possible to the right. Inhale deeply.

2 With an exhalation, twist and bend your body from the waist. Place your left hand either flat on the floor outside your right foot or on top of your right ankle. Raise your right arm straight upward and look up at it. Breathe rhythmically, holding for up to 1 minute, then repeat on the opposite side. Follow with final relaxation (see pp192–193).

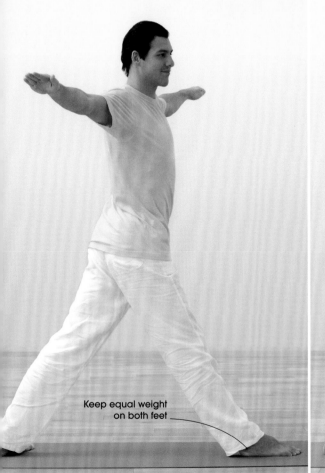

Keep equal weight on both feet

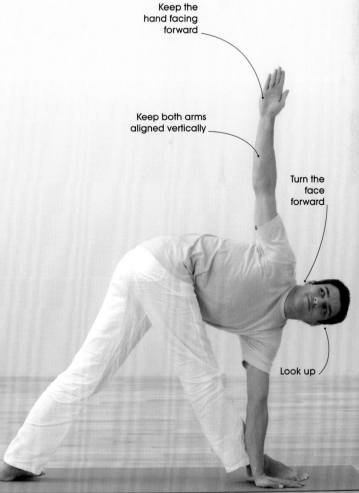

Keep the hand facing forward

Keep both arms aligned vertically

Turn the face forward

Look up

Triangle
Variations (continued)

These variations give special attention to stretching and strengthening the pelvic girdle. The isometric contraction of the quadriceps muscles provides an intense workout for the thighs.

Triangle with Bent Knee Intermediate

1 Stand with your legs farther apart than in Triangle Step 1 (see p164). Turn your left foot to the left, bend your left knee, and rest your left forearm on it. Keep your right leg straight. Breathe rhythmically.

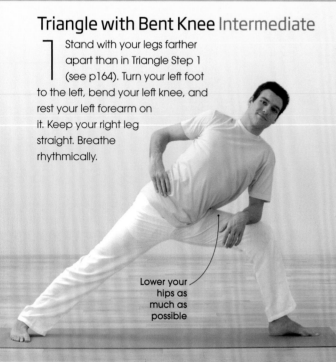

Lower your hips as much as possible

2 Turn your torso to the left, exhale, and place both palms on the floor, parallel to each other, and to the inside of your left foot.

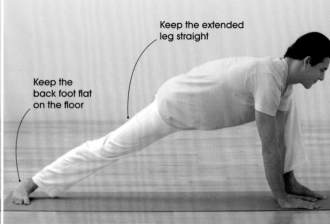

Keep the extended leg straight

Keep the back foot flat on the floor

3 Inhale and lift your right arm, taking it alongside your right ear. Hold for up to 30 seconds, breathing rhythmically. To come out of the pose, lift your left arm straight up and, with a push of your left leg, stand up straight again. Repeat on the opposite side. Follow with final relaxation (see pp192–193).

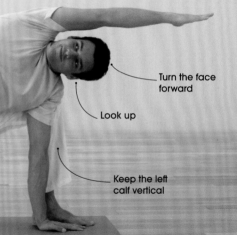

Keep the back foot flat on the floor

Turn the face forward

Look up

Keep the left calf vertical

Head to Toe
Advanced

4 Starting from Triangle with Bent Knee Step 2 (see opposite), take your hands behind your back and interlock your fingers. Inhale and lift your back until it is aligned with your left leg, keeping your balance on both feet.

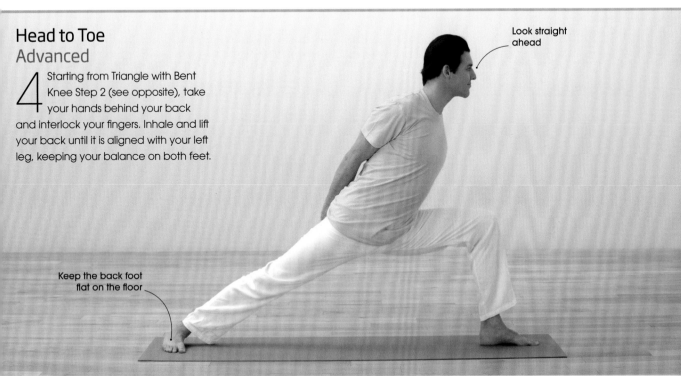

Look straight ahead

Keep the back foot flat on the floor

5 Exhale, bend forward, and try to place the top of your head on the floor next to your left foot. Hold for up to 30 seconds. With an inhalation, come out of the pose by lifting your torso, then repeat on the opposite side. Follow with final relaxation (see pp192–193).

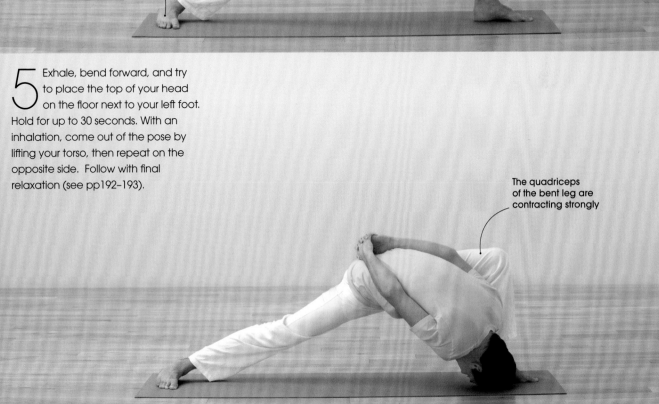

The quadriceps of the bent leg are contracting strongly

Sequences

The sequences in this section offer routines suitable for beginner, intermediate, and advanced levels; at each level there is a 20-, 40-, and 60-minute sequence. Remember to always rest in Corpse Pose (see p46) before you begin.

Beginner's Sequences

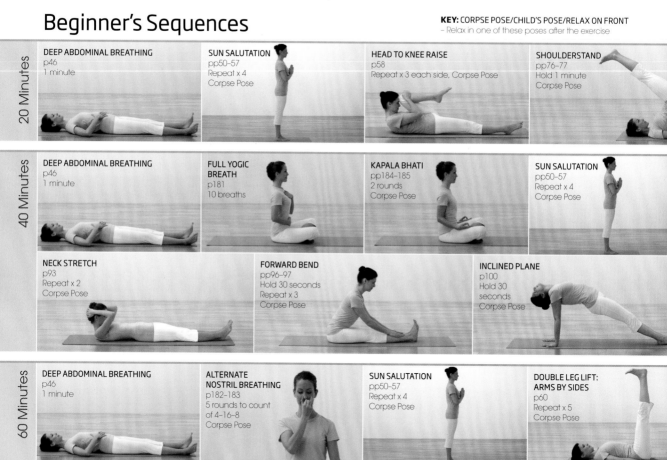

20 Minutes

DEEP ABDOMINAL BREATHING
p46
1 minute

SUN SALUTATION
pp50–57
Repeat x 4
Corpse Pose

HEAD TO KNEE RAISE
p58
Repeat x 3 each side, Corpse Pose

SHOULDERSTAND
pp76–77
Hold 1 minute
Corpse Pose

40 Minutes

DEEP ABDOMINAL BREATHING
p46
1 minute

FULL YOGIC BREATH
p181
10 breaths

KAPALA BHATI
pp184–185
2 rounds
Corpse Pose

SUN SALUTATION
pp50–57
Repeat x 4
Corpse Pose

NECK STRETCH
p93
Repeat x 2
Corpse Pose

FORWARD BEND
pp96–97
Hold 30 seconds
Repeat x 3
Corpse Pose

INCLINED PLANE
p100
Hold 30 seconds
Corpse Pose

60 Minutes

DEEP ABDOMINAL BREATHING
p46
1 minute

ALTERNATE NOSTRIL BREATHING
p182–183
5 rounds to count of 4–16–8
Corpse Pose

SUN SALUTATION
pp50–57
Repeat x 4
Corpse Pose

DOUBLE LEG LIFT: ARMS BY SIDES
p60
Repeat x 5
Corpse Pose

SHOULDERSTAND
pp76–77
Hold 1 minute
Corpse Pose

BRIDGE
p86
Hold 30 seconds
Corpse Pose

FISH
pp92–93
Hold 1 minute

NECK STRETCH
p93
Repeat x 2
Corpse Pose

COBRA
pp116–117
Hold 5 breaths
Repeat x 3
Relax on front

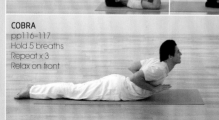

LOCUST
pp122–123
Hold 20 seconds each leg
Relax on front

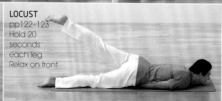

BOW
p134
Hold 20 seconds each side
Relax on front, then Child's Pose

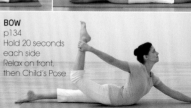

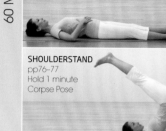
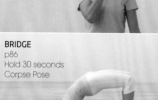
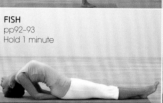
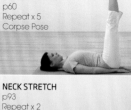

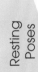

Resting Poses

CORPSE POSE p46, 8 breaths between poses, 6–10 minutes in Final Relaxation (see pp192–193)

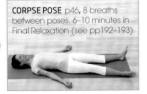

CHILD'S POSE p191
8 breaths after backward bends

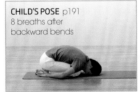

RELAX ON FRONT p190
8 breaths after backward bends

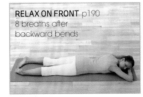

PLOUGH WITH FEET APART
p84
Hold 1 minute
Corpse Pose

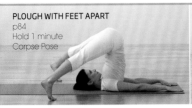

FISH
pp92–93
Hold 30 seconds

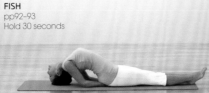

NECK STRETCH
p93
Repeat x 2
Final relaxation, about 6 minutes

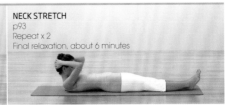

SINGLE LEG LIFT
p58
Repeat x 6
each side
Corpse Pose

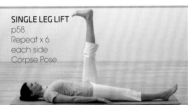

SHOULDERSTAND
pp76–77
Hold 1 minute
Corpse Pose

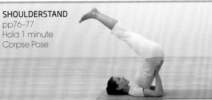

FISH
pp92–93
Hold 1 minute

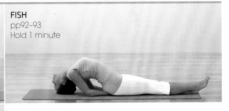

CAMEL
p128
Hold up to
30 seconds
Child's Pose

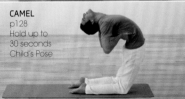

TRIANGLE
pp164–165
Hold 20 seconds
each side
Corpse Pose
Final Relaxation
10 minutes

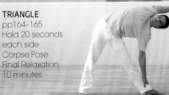

DOLPHIN
pp62–63
Repeat x 4
Child's Pose

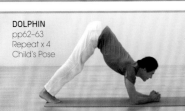

SHOULDERSTAND
pp76–77
Hold 1 minute

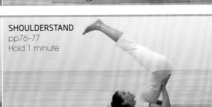

PLOUGH WITH FEET APART
p84
Hold 1 minute

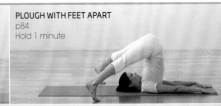

SINGLE LEG FORWARD BEND
p102
Hold 1 minute each side

FORWARD BEND
pp96–97
Hold 1 minute
Repeat x 2

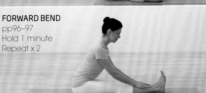

INCLINED PLANE
p100
Hold 30
seconds
Corpse Pose

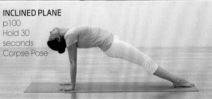

HALF SPINAL TWIST
pp144–145
Hold 30 seconds
each side
Child's Pose

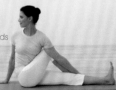

TREE
p158
Hold 20 seconds
each side

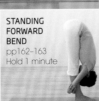

STANDING FORWARD BEND
pp162–163
Hold 1 minute

TRIANGLE
pp164–165
Hold 20 seconds
each side
Final relaxation
10 minutes

Intermediate Sequences

KEY: CORPSE POSE/CHILD'S POSE/RELAX ON FRONT – Relax in one of these poses after the exercise

Resting Poses

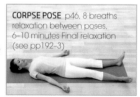

CORPSE POSE p46, 8 breaths relaxation between poses, 6–10 minutes Final relaxation (see pp192–3)

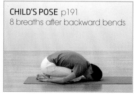

CHILD'S POSE p191 8 breaths after backward bends

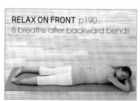

RELAX ON FRONT p190 8 breaths after backward bends

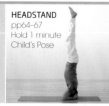

HEADSTAND pp64–67 Hold 1 minute Child's Pose

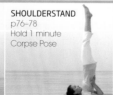

SHOULDERSTAND p76–78 Hold 1 minute Corpse Pose

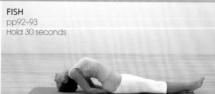

FISH pp92–93 Hold 30 seconds

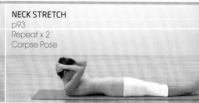

NECK STRETCH p93 Repeat x 2 Corpse Pose

---

40 Minutes

KAPALA BHATI pp184–185 1 round

ALTERNATE NOSTRIL BREATHING p182 4 rounds to count of 5-20-10 Corpse Pose

SUN SALUTATION pp50–57 Repeat x 6 Corpse Pose

DEEP STRETCH SINGLE LEG LIFT pp58–59 Hold 30 seconds each side, Corpse Pose

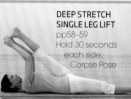

FORWARD BEND: WITH WIDE LEGS p104 Hold 1 minute

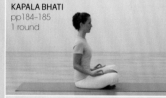

FORWARD BEND pp96–99 Hold 1 minute

INCLINED PLANE p100 Hold 30 seconds

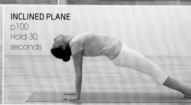

---

60 Minutes

KAPALA BHATI pp184–185 3 rounds

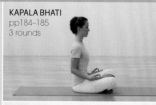

ALTERNATE NOSTRIL BREATHING pp182–183 5 rounds count of 5-20-10 Corpse Pose

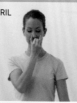

SUN SALUTATION pp50–57 Repeat x 10 Corpse Pose

HEADSTAND: KNEES BENT TO THE SIDES p69 Hold 1 minute Child's Pose

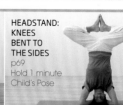

FISH pp92–93 Hold 1 minute Corpse Pose

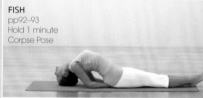

SHOOTING BOW p110 Hold 30 seconds each side

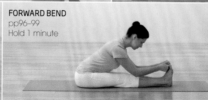

FORWARD BEND pp96–99 Hold 2 minutes

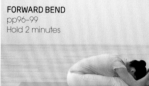

BOW: ROCKING BOW p136 Rock 8 times back and forth Child's Pose

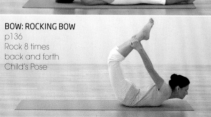

HALF SPINAL TWIST: WRIST GRASP p148 Hold 1 minute each side Child's Pose

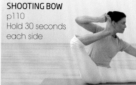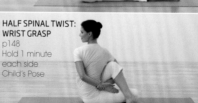

STANDING FORWARD BEND pp162–163 Hold 1 minute

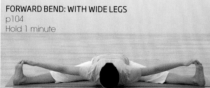

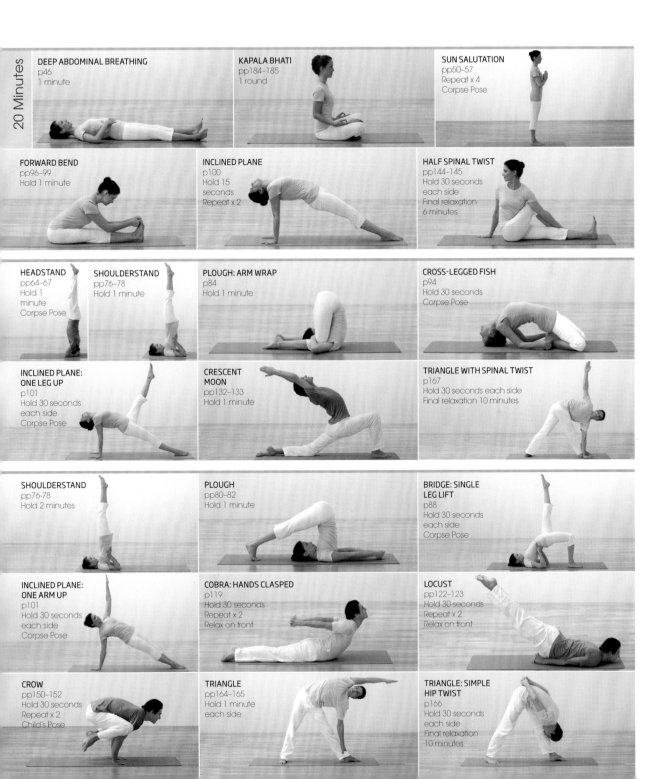

20 Minutes

DEEP ABDOMINAL BREATHING
p46
1 minute

KAPALA BHATI
pp184–185
1 round

SUN SALUTATION
pp50–57
Repeat x 4
Corpse Pose

FORWARD BEND
pp96–99
Hold 1 minute

INCLINED PLANE
p100
Hold 15
seconds
Repeat x 2

HALF SPINAL TWIST
pp144–145
Hold 30 seconds
each side
Final relaxation
6 minutes

HEADSTAND
pp64–67
Hold 1
minute
Corpse Pose

SHOULDERSTAND
pp76–78
Hold 1 minute

PLOUGH: ARM WRAP
p84
Hold 1 minute

CROSS-LEGGED FISH
p94
Hold 30 seconds
Corpse Pose

**INCLINED PLANE:
ONE LEG UP**
p101
Hold 30 seconds
each side
Corpse Pose

**CRESCENT
MOON**
pp132–133
Hold 1 minute

TRIANGLE WITH SPINAL TWIST
p167
Hold 30 seconds each side
Final relaxation 10 minutes

SHOULDERSTAND
pp76–78
Hold 2 minutes

PLOUGH
pp80–82
Hold 1 minute

**BRIDGE: SINGLE
LEG LIFT**
p88
Hold 30 seconds
each side
Corpse Pose

**INCLINED PLANE:
ONE ARM UP**
p101
Hold 30 seconds
each side
Corpse Pose

COBRA: HANDS CLASPED
p119
Hold 30 seconds
Repeat x 2
Relax on front

LOCUST
pp122–123
Hold 30 seconds
Repeat x 2
Relax on front

CROW
pp150–152
Hold 30 seconds
Repeat x 2
Child's Pose

TRIANGLE
pp164–165
Hold 1 minute
each side

**TRIANGLE: SIMPLE
HIP TWIST**
p166
Hold 30 seconds
each side
Final relaxation
10 minutes

Advanced Sequences

KEY: CORPSE POSE/CHILD'S POSE/RELAX ON FRONT – *Relax in one of these poses after the exercise*

Resting Poses

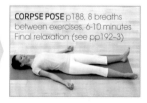

CORPSE POSE p188, 8 breaths between exercises, 6-10 minutes Final relaxation (see pp192-3)

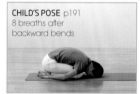

CHILD'S POSE p191 8 breaths after backward bends

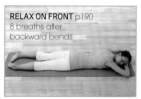

RELAX ON FRONT p190 8 breaths after backward bends

PLOUGH: ARM WRAP
p84
Hold 30 seconds

PLOUGH: KNEES BEHIND HEAD
p85
Hold 30 seconds

LOTUS FISH
p95
Hold 30 seconds
Corpse Pose

---

40 Minutes

KAPALA BHATI
pp184-185
2 rounds

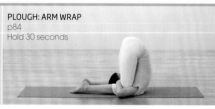

SUN SALUTATION
pp50-57
Repeat x 6
Corpse Pose

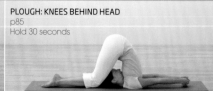

LOTUS HEADSTAND
p70
Hold 1 minute

TWISTED LOTUS HEADSTAND
p71
Hold 15 seconds each side

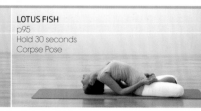

FORWARD BEND
pp96-99
Hold 2 minutes
Corpse Pose

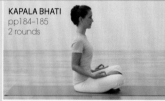

CRESCENT SPLITS
p112-113
Hold 30 seconds each side

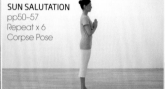

KING COBRA
pp120-121
Hold 30 seconds

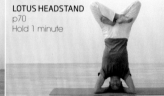

ROCKING BOW
p136
Practise 30 seconds
Child's Pose

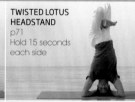

---

60 Minutes

KAPALA BHATI
pp184-185
3 rounds

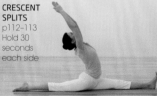

ALTERNATE NOSTRIL BREATHING
p182-183
5 rounds to count of 6-24-12
Corpse Pose

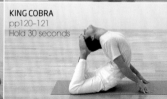

SUN SALUTATION
pp50-57
Repeat x 8
Corpse Pose

HEADSTAND
pp64-67
Hold 3 minutes
Child's Pose

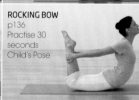

LOTUS FISH
p95
Hold 2 minutes
Corpse Pose

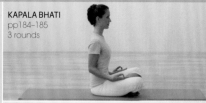

STRAIGHT ARM FORWARD BEND
p105
Hold 3 minutes

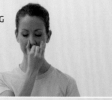

LATERAL BEND WITH TWIST
p107
Hold 1 minute each side

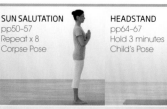

FULL SPINAL TWIST
p149
Hold 30 seconds each side

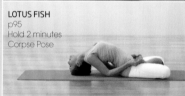

LOTUS PEACOCK
p157
Hold 1 minute

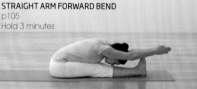

DANCING LORD SIVA
pp160-161
Hold 1 minute each side

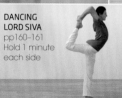

TRIANGLE: HEAD TO TOE
p169
Hold 1 minute each side
Final relaxation
8 minutes

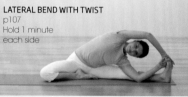
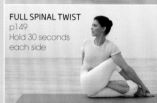
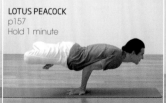
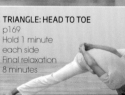

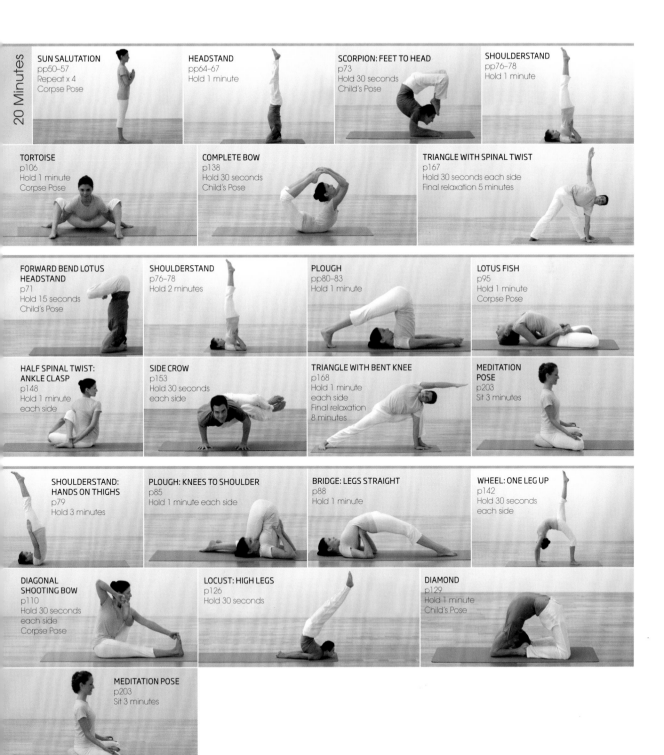

20 Minutes

SUN SALUTATION
pp50–57
Repeat x 4
Corpse Pose

HEADSTAND
pp64–67
Hold 1 minute

SCORPION: FEET TO HEAD
p73
Hold 30 seconds
Child's Pose

SHOULDERSTAND
pp76–78
Hold 1 minute

TORTOISE
p106
Hold 1 minute
Corpse Pose

COMPLETE BOW
p138
Hold 30 seconds
Child's Pose

TRIANGLE WITH SPINAL TWIST
p167
Hold 30 seconds each side
Final relaxation 5 minutes

FORWARD BEND LOTUS HEADSTAND
p71
Hold 15 seconds
Child's Pose

SHOULDERSTAND
p76–78
Hold 2 minutes

PLOUGH
pp80–83
Hold 1 minute

LOTUS FISH
p95
Hold 1 minute
Corpse Pose

HALF SPINAL TWIST: ANKLE CLASP
p148
Hold 1 minute
each side

SIDE CROW
p153
Hold 30 seconds
each side

TRIANGLE WITH BENT KNEE
p168
Hold 1 minute
each side
Final relaxation
8 minutes

MEDITATION POSE
p203
Sit 3 minutes

SHOULDERSTAND: HANDS ON THIGHS
p79
Hold 3 minutes

PLOUGH: KNEES TO SHOULDER
p85
Hold 1 minute each side

BRIDGE: LEGS STRAIGHT
p88
Hold 1 minute

WHEEL: ONE LEG UP
p142
Hold 30 seconds
each side

DIAGONAL SHOOTING BOW
p110
Hold 30 seconds
each side
Corpse Pose

LOCUST: HIGH LEGS
p126
Hold 30 seconds

DIAMOND
p129
Hold 1 minute
Child's Pose

MEDITATION POSE
p203
Sit 3 minutes

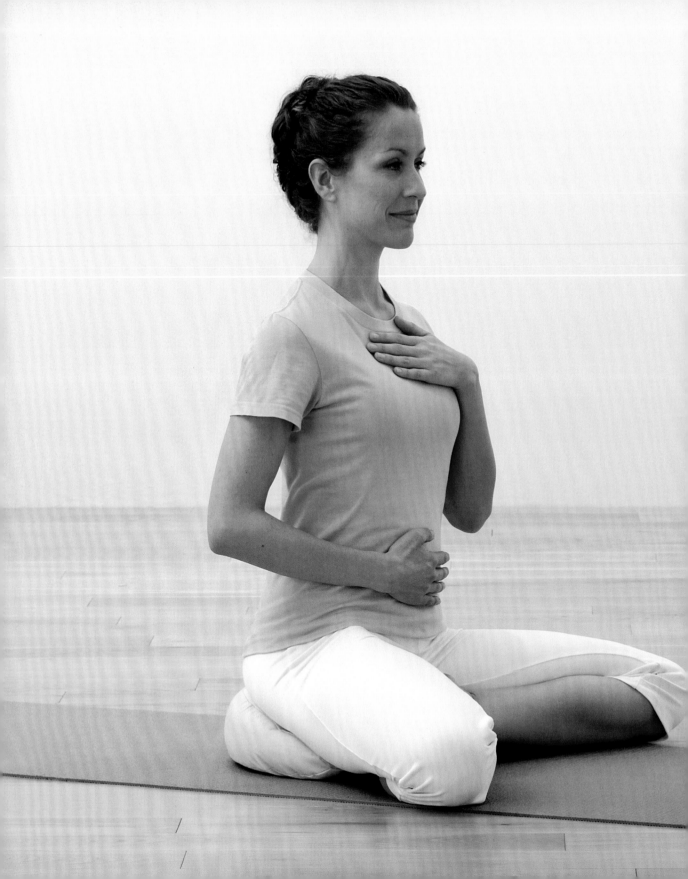

Proper
Breathing

Pranayama

In the yogic tradition, the breath is seen as the outward manifestation of prana, or vital energy. Gaining control of the breath by practicing breathing exercises—pranayama— increases the flow of prana through the body, which literally recharges body and mind. Aim to practice pranayama for up to 30 minutes daily, before or after asana practice.

Circulation of prana

According to the ancient yogic texts, prana circulates through the body in a network of 72,000 astral energy channels, or *nadis*. These not only permeate every part of the body, but also create an extensive energy field, or aura, around it. When you perform asanas, you apply pressure to points where important nadis cross. This works like acupressure, unblocking vital energy.

Strengthening the flow of prana

Yoga breathing exercises focus specifically on opening two major nadis—the *pingala* nadi and the *ida nadi*—and strengthening the flow of prana in them. The pingala nadi corresponds to the right nostril and left hemisphere of the brain, and the ida nadi to the left nostril and right brain. In the mystical language of yoga, the pingala nadi is warming and corresponds to "*Ha*" or the sun; the ida is cooling and corresponds to "*Tha*" or the moon. The final step of the eight-fold path of Hatha and Raja Yoga (see p11) comes about when there is perfect balance between these two nadis. The most important nadi, however, is the *sushumna*, which corresponds to the spinal cord. When the pingala and ida nadis are in balance, the sushumna opens, allowing vital energy to flow upward and spiritual enlightenment to occur.

Training the respiratory muscles

Although the language and imagery of pranayama may appear quite mystical, in practice its effects are concrete. Whether you are a beginner or a more advanced yoga practitioner, pranayama trains the respiratory muscles, develops use of your lungs' full capacity, and improves your body's supply of oxygen while reducing its carbon dioxide levels. It also helps to relax and strengthen your nervous system, calm the mind, and improve concentration.

Begin your pranayama practice by lying in Corpse Pose (see p46) for 2–3 minutes. After your practice, relax in Corpse Pose again to release any tension in the hips or lower back from sitting in a cross-legged position.

What is prana?

Prana, or vital energy, is found in all forms of life, from mineral to mankind, where its force controls and regulates every part of the body. Although prana is in all forms of matter, it is not matter. It is the energy that animates matter.

Prana is in the air, but it is not oxygen, nor any of its chemical constituents. It is in food, water, and sunlight, and yet it is not vitamin, heat, or light. Food, water, and air are only the media through which prana is carried. We absorb prana through the food we eat, the water we drink, and the air we breathe.

The easiest way to control prana is to regulate the breath—pranayama. Every part of the body can be filled with prana and when we do this, the entire body is under our control.

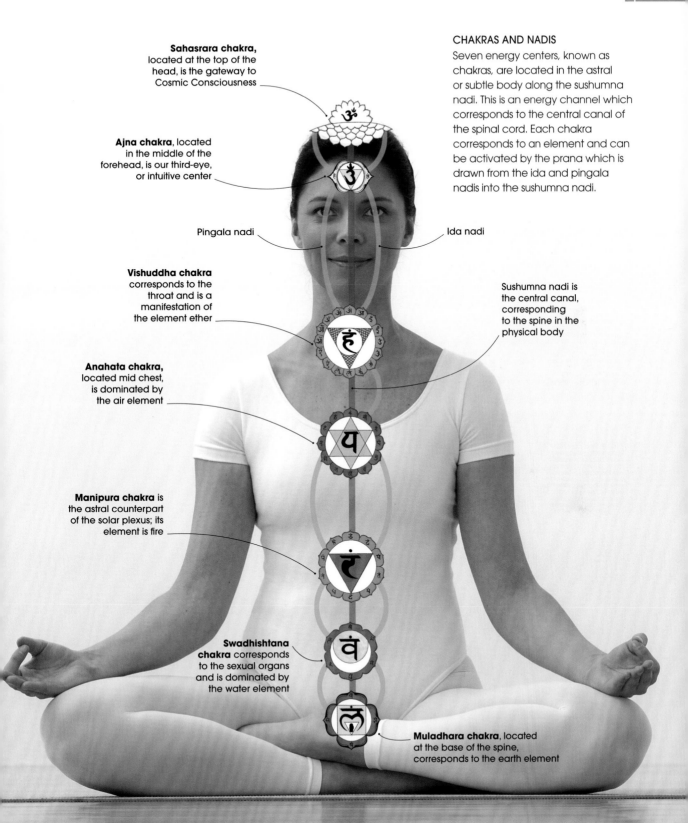

Sahasrara chakra, located at the top of the head, is the gateway to Cosmic Consciousness

Ajna chakra, located in the middle of the forehead, is our third-eye, or intuitive center

Pingala nadi

Vishuddha chakra corresponds to the throat and is a manifestation of the element ether

Anahata chakra, located mid chest, is dominated by the air element

Manipura chakra is the astral counterpart of the solar plexus; its element is fire

Swadhishtana chakra corresponds to the sexual organs and is dominated by the water element

CHAKRAS AND NADIS

Seven energy centers, known as chakras, are located in the astral or subtle body along the sushumna nadi. This is an energy channel which corresponds to the central canal of the spinal cord. Each chakra corresponds to an element and can be activated by the prana which is drawn from the ida and pingala nadis into the sushumna nadi.

Ida nadi

Sushumna nadi is the central canal, corresponding to the spine in the physical body

Muladhara chakra, located at the base of the spine, corresponds to the earth element

Preparatory exercises

Abdominal Breathing is the essential preparatory technique to master before beginning any pranayama exercise. This is the first stage on the road to the Full Yogic Breath, which teaches you how to make full use of your lungs' capacity. Once you can comfortably practice this, you are ready for the pranayama exercises on pp182–185.

Abdominal Breathing

Learning how to breathe deeply using your abdomen is one of the keys to pranayama. Practice it first when you relax in Corpse Pose (see p46) in preparation for your asana practice, and repeat it when you lie in Corpse Pose before your pranayama session. For several minutes, focus on slow, rhythmical breathing and the movement of your abdomen.

During Abdominal Breathing, the diaphragm draws air into and expels it from the lowest—and largest—part of the lungs. In order for the diaphragm to move freely, your abdominal muscles must be completely relaxed, so practice for a few minutes.

"If your body is strong and healthy with much prana, you will have a natural tendency to produce health and vitality in those close to you.

Swami Vishnudevananda

Practicing Abdominal Breathing

Lie in Corpse Pose (see p46), palms on your abdomen and fingers apart. As you breathe, feel the movement between your first rib, your navel, and your hips. Notice movement in the back of your body, too, around the kidneys and the lower back, and below your waist.

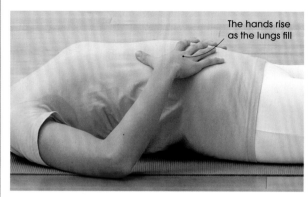

The hands rise
as the lungs fill

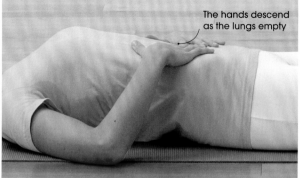

The hands descend
as the lungs empty

INHALATION
Inhale for five seconds. As your abdomen expands, notice how your hands rise and your fingers draw apart.

EXHALATION
Exhale for five seconds. Notice your hands moving down and fingers coming together. Repeat the in and out breaths for two minutes.

Full Yogic Breath

This complete breath makes full use of your respiratory muscles. Learning to fill and empty the lungs to their maximum in a relaxed and controlled manner has a multitude of uses. It improves your muscle strength as you move into, hold, and release an asana. And when you perform a few cycles of the Full Yogic Breath during the short relaxation period between one asana and the next, it helps quickly to replenish the oxygen you have used while practicing the asana. The muscle control you develop in the Full Yogic Breath—from the pelvis right up to the skull—also improves your awareness of spinal alignment in an asana. You might like to perform a few full yogic breaths as a quick pick-me-up at work, too, to help replenish your energy levels and quickly restore concentration.

Practicing Full Yogic Breath

Positioning your hands on your abdomen and chest helps you learn to contract and relax the respiratory muscles in the correct order. If you find it easier, begin with a few breaths in Corpse Pose (see p46) before sitting up. Breathe very slowly throughout.

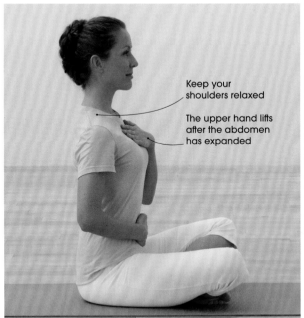

Keep your shoulders relaxed

The upper hand lifts after the abdomen has expanded

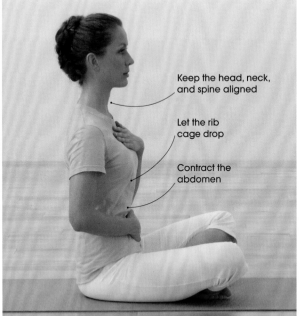

Keep the head, neck, and spine aligned

Let the rib cage drop

Contract the abdomen

INHALATION
Sit in a comfortable, cross-legged position and place one hand on your chest and the other on your abdomen. As you inhale, gradually expand the abdomen, then raise and open the rib cage, and finally lift the collarbone.

EXHALATION
Begin the exhalation by relaxing the abdomen, then lower the rib cage, and finally slightly contract the abdomen to actively empty the lungs. Repeat the inhalations and exhalations in this way for about two minutes.

Alternate Nostril Breathing

This is an excellent exercise for balancing the nervous system. Practicing it can calm you down when you feel hyperactive, stimulate you when you feel lethargic, and center you when you feel distracted. The prolonged exhalations release tension, the deep inhalations draw prana into the solar plexus, and, when you retain the breath, prana is directed to the area of the third eye, bringing about mental poise.

How to practice

Pranayama should feel pleasant and never stressful. Beginners will find the ratio of inhalation to retention and exhalation in the complete technique too challenging, so start with Single Nostril Breathing before progressing through the levels. You will feel the benefits, no matter which level you practice.

Single Nostril Breathing

Place your right hand in front of your face in Vishnu Mudra (see below, right). Close your right nostril with your thumb (see opposite). Inhale for three seconds and exhale for six seconds through your left nostril. This is one round. Practice up to 10 rounds. Repeat on the other nostril: close your left nostril with your ring finger and inhale and exhale through your right nostril. Practice 10 rounds on each side regularly over a few weeks. Gradually increase the ratio of the exhalation to the inhalation—first inhale for four seconds and exhale for eight, then lengthen the ratio to 5:10, and finally to 6:12.

Simple Alternate Nostril Breathing

After mastering the 6:12 ratio of Single Nostril Breathing, move on to simple Alternate Nostril Breathing. Closing your right nostril with your thumb, inhale through your left nostril for four seconds, close your left nostril with your ring finger, open your right nostril and exhale through it for eight seconds. Inhale through your right nostril for four seconds, then exhale through your left nostril for eight seconds. Practice up to 10 rounds. Gradually increase the inhalation:exhalation ratio to 5:10, then to 6:12, and finally to 7:14.

Alternate Nostril Breathing with Retention

Once you have mastered the 7:14 ratio of the simple Alternate Nostril Breathing, move on to Alternate Nostril Breathing with Breath Retention. Inhale through your left nostril for four seconds, close the nostril (see opposite), hold your breath for eight seconds, then exhale through your

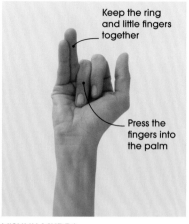

VISHNU MUDRA
Hold your right hand with the palm facing you and fold the first and second fingers into the palm. Try to keep your thumb and ring and little fingers straight.

Keep the ring and little fingers together

Press the fingers into the palm

Positioning the hand

Using a *mudra*, or energetic seal, like Vishnu Mudra (see opposite) helps to contain prana within the body, but is useful on a purely physical level, too, providing a tangible aid to concentration.

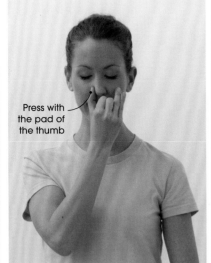

Press with the pad of the thumb

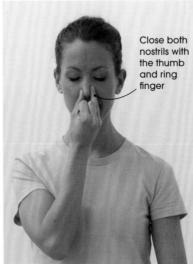

Close both nostrils with the thumb and ring finger

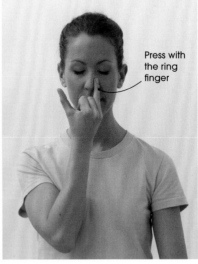

Press with the ring finger

BREATHING THROUGH THE LEFT NOSTRIL
With your right hand in Vishnu Mudra (see opposite), close the right nostril with your thumb; inhale through the left nostril.

BREATH RETENTION
To retain your breath, close both nostrils with the thumb and the ring finger.

BREATHING THROUGH THE RIGHT NOSTRIL
Close the left nostril with your ring finger, and exhale through the right nostril.

right nostril for eight seconds. Then inhale through your right nostril for four seconds, hold your breath for eight seconds and exhale through your left nostril for eight seconds. Practice up to 10 rounds. Increase the inhalation:retention:exhalation ratio to 5:10:10, then to 6:12:12, and finally to 7:14:14.

Complete Alternate Nostril Breathing

As you improve, try a longer breath retention—complete Alternate Nostril Breathing. Inhale through your left nostril for four seconds, hold the breath for 16 seconds, and exhale through the right nostril for eight seconds. Then inhale through the right nostril for four seconds, hold the breath for 16 seconds, and exhale through the left nostril for eight seconds. Practice up to 10 rounds. Increase the inhalation:retention:exhalation ratio to 5:20:10, then to 6:24:12, and finally to 7:28:14.

Kapala Bhati

Literally translated as "shining skull," this exercise cleanses the respiratory passages, including the nasal passages in the head. It is one of the kriyas, or organ-cleansing exercises of Hatha and Raja Yoga (see pp10–11). Kapala Bhati also increases the capacity of the lungs, stimulates blood circulation, and gives a gentle massage to the heart. People who have asthma often find it helpful.

How to practice

Kapala Bhati consists of a series of short and active exhalations, alternated with passive, relaxed inhalations. The intense expulsions of stale air from the lungs increase the uptake of oxygen into the blood, which can be felt especially in the brain. This makes Kapala Bhati an excellent way to improve your concentration, whether you are practicing meditation or need a quick mental boost at work.

This exercise is best practiced during a morning pranayama or meditation session; do not practice it late in the evening, since it activates the nervous system and may prevent you from falling asleep. If you are a beginner, do not try Kapala Bhati until you feel completely at ease practicing Alternate Nostril Breathing with Breath Retention (see pp182–183).

Intermediate level

Sit with your legs crossed and your hands in Chin Mudra (see p204) and take a few slow, deep abdominal breaths. Notice the abdomen moving out as you inhale and in as you exhale. Then start a series of 10 rhythmic, short, active exhalations (see opposite). After each active exhalation, let a gentle, passive in-breath just happen (see opposite). The time taken for one exhalation and inhalation should be about two seconds.

After 10 of these "pumps" out and in, take two slow full yogic breaths (see p181). Then inhale comfortably to 80 percent of your capacity and hold the breath, according to your ability, for 20–60 seconds. Exhale slowly, with control. This is one round. After a few relaxed breaths, practice two more rounds.

Advanced level

Using the same technique, gradually increase the number of times you "pump" out and in per round to 50. You can speed up the rate at which you breathe, but never faster than one second for one exhalation and inhalation. As you become more relaxed and focused, try to hold the breath during the

---

Avoiding hyperventilation

When you practice Kapala Bhati for the first time, you may feel dizzy. This is caused by hyperventilation. If this happens, stop immediately, lie on your back and relax. Once the dizziness has gone, check whether you were making one of the following mistakes, and take the remedying action set out below.

The chest or collarbone move: Check that only your abdomen is moving during both exhalations and inhalations.

Your abdomen is not moving in when you exhale: Check that your abdomen is actively contracting and moving inward every time you exhale.

You are inhaling too deeply or you are actively pushing out your abdomen: Inhale passively so that the abdomen simply moves forward into its neutral position.

You are pumping too fast: Reduce the speed of the pumping to two seconds for one inhalation and exhalation.

retention for up to 90 seconds. While you are holding your breath, focus on the third-eye area between your eyebrows. While you hold your breath, you may feel a pleasant warmth around your abdomen. This is the activated prana in your solar plexus. With each round of practice, the solar plexus recharges further, and prana starts moving up the spine. After sustained practice, you will find that the movement of prana is in accordance with how focused you are. The energy literally moves to where your thoughts go, which is why you should focus on the third eye.

Inhaling and exhaling

It is important to get the "pumping" technique right in this powerful exercise. Emphasize the exhalation; if you do this correctly, it creates a vacuum and the in-breath happens naturally, without requiring any effort.

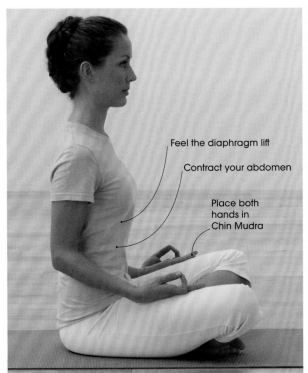

Feel the diaphragm lift

Contract your abdomen

Place both hands in Chin Mudra

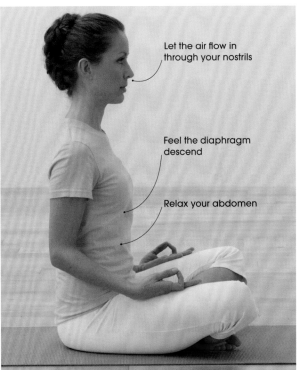

Let the air flow in through your nostrils

Feel the diaphragm descend

Relax your abdomen

ACTIVE EXHALATION
To actively exhale, firmly contract your abdomen and feel your diaphragm lift to push the air out of your lungs forcefully through both nostrils.

PASSIVE INHALATION
To inhale passively, simply release the abdomen. Feel the diaphragm descend and the air rush in. Do not try to take a breath; let the inhalation come easily, by itself.

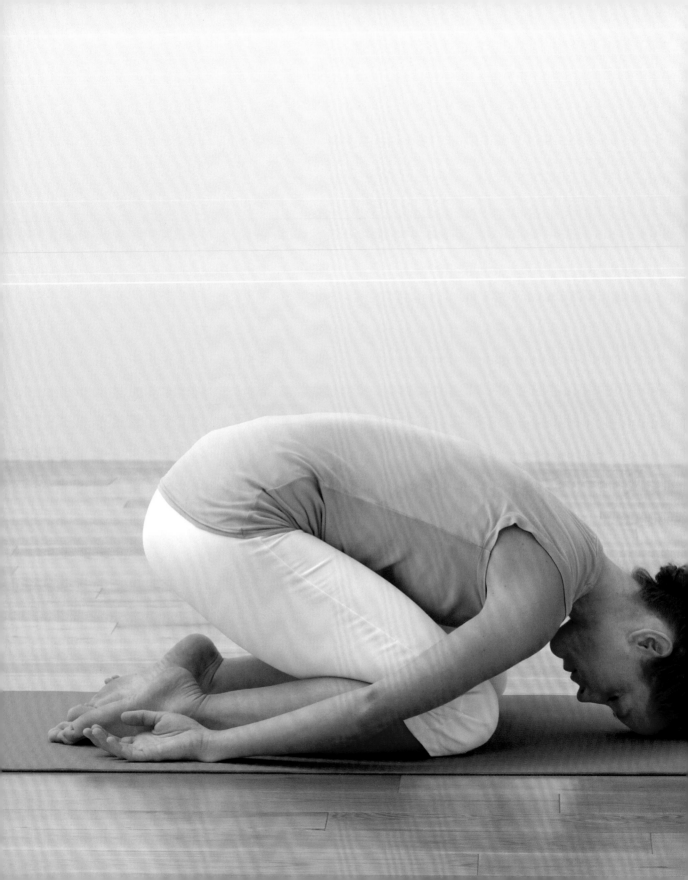

Proper
Relaxation

Relaxation between asanas

Take time to relax between one asana and the next—this allows the body to absorb the effects of the pose and be reinvigorated. Relax for a minimum of 8 deep breaths, but for no more than 2 minutes, so the body stays warm to progress to the next pose.

Why relax?

When you are performing postures, you can observe how the asana practice contains its own, inbuilt rhythmical alternation between effort and relaxation. In some asanas, your muscles are first stretched and then relaxed; in others, they are contracted and then relaxed (see p36). Relaxing between asanas confirms this pattern of effort and release in your nervous system, so that by the time you reach the final relaxation (see pp192–193), your nervous system is so well balanced that you will be able to relax simply by visualizing yourself relaxed—in other words, by using autosuggestion (see p194).

Relaxing on your back

Corpse Pose is the preferred position for relaxation between most asanas— exceptions are for backward bends and inversions. If you find this pose uncomfortable, use the alternative pose on the opposite page.

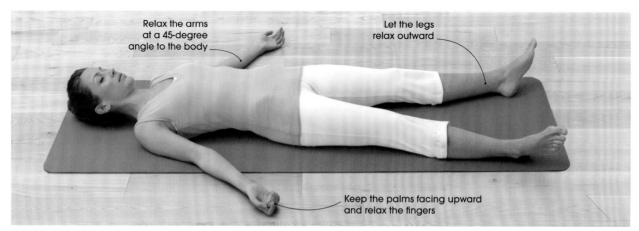

Relax the arms at a 45-degree angle to the body

Let the legs relax outward

Keep the palms facing upward and relax the fingers

CORPSE POSE

To get into Corpse Pose, follow the instructions for the initial relaxation. Take at least 8 deep, rhythmical breaths as you lie in Corpse Pose, and notice the effects of the pose you have just completed on your body and mind. Then progress to the next asana. If you find Corpse Pose uncomfortable, try the alternative positions opposite.

Alternative supine position

You may be uncomfortable lying on your back if you are unable to relax the muscles of the lower back fully. If this is the case, try the exercise below. After some practice, you will find that you can lie more comfortably in Corpse Pose to relax between asanas.

> ## When Corpse Pose is uncomfortable
>
> Bringing your knees toward your chest releases tension in the lower back. You can then drop your feet to the floor and practice the relaxation between asanas with your knees bent and your feet hip-width apart.
>
>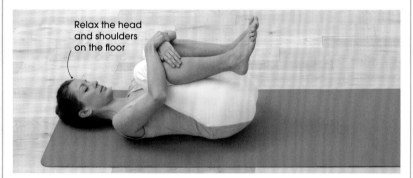
>
> Relax the head and shoulders on the floor
>
> **HUGGING THE KNEES**
> Bend both legs and bring your knees toward your chest. Wrap your arms around your knees, and hold onto one wrist with the other hand. This gives the lower back a gentle stretch and releases tension around that part of the spine.
>
>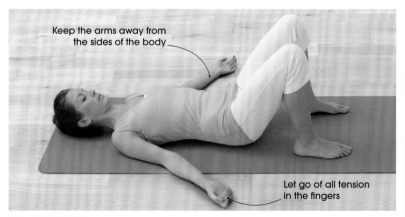
>
> Keep the arms away from the sides of the body
>
> Let go of all tension in the fingers
>
> **FEET ON FLOOR**
> Place your feet flat on the floor, about 8in (20cm) from your buttocks and relax your arms to the sides, with the palms facing upward and the fingers completely relaxed. Take at least 8 deep, rhythmical breaths before progressing to the next asana.

"In order to regulate and balance the work of the body and mind, it is necessary to economize the energy produced by the body. This is the main purpose of learning how to relax."

Swami Vishnudevananda

Relaxing on your front

After asanas such as Cobra (see pp116–121) and Locust (see pp122–123), and variations performed from a prone position—lying on your abdomen—relax on your front before moving on to the next asana (see below). As you relax, notice the effect of the pose you have just performed on your body and mind, and feel the respiratory movement in your abdomen.

Relaxing on your abdomen

Turning your legs in these prone relaxation positions creates rotation in the hip joints, which helps the muscles in the legs to relax. If your body feels tense or you get cramps in the feet in the basic position, try the alternative position (see below).

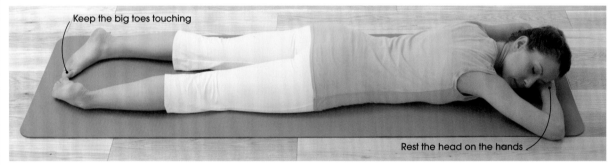

Keep the big toes touching

Rest the head on the hands

BASIC POSITION
Lie on your front with your arms folded in front of you and your hands one on top of the other. Turn your head to one side and rest it on your hands. This releases tension in the neck and shoulders and makes breathing more comfortable. The "pillow" formed by your hands takes any pressure away from your cheeks. Keep your legs slightly apart and turn your toes inward. Take at least 8 deep, rhythmical breaths before progressing to the next asana.

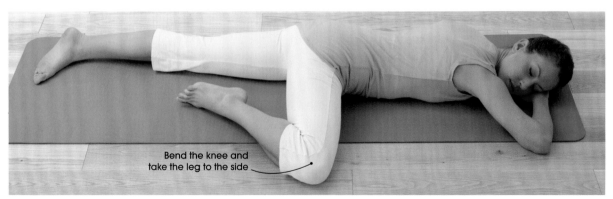

Bend the knee and take the leg to the side

ALTERNATIVE POSITION
Lie on your front with your arms folded in front of your head and your hands one on top of the other. Turn your head to one side and rest it on your hands. Keep your legs slightly apart and turn your toes inward. Bend one knee and take the leg out to the side, toward your arm—this is Baby Krishna Pose. Keep your extended leg, your spine, and your head aligned. Take at least 8 deep, rhythmical breaths before progressing to the next asana.

Following Headstand (see pp62–75), Half Spinal Twist (see pp144–149), and any backward-bending asanas, relax in Child's Pose (see below). Child's Pose is good for relaxing the head and shoulders and gently stretching out the spine, which invigorates the nervous system. This pose also brings a refreshing flow of blood to the brain, for a rejuvenating effect before you move on to practice the next pose.

Relaxing in a forward bend

The slight forward bend in Child's Pose gives your back and the muscles around your hips a soothing stretch. If you find it difficult to sit on your heels or your forehead does not reach the floor, practice the variation (see below).

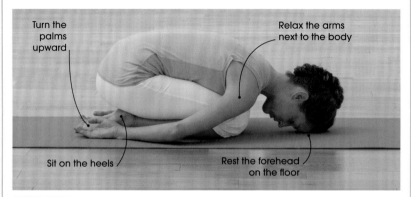

Turn the palms upward
Relax the arms next to the body
Sit on the heels
Rest the forehead on the floor

CHILD POSE
Sit on your heels and lean forward until your forehead comes to the floor. Extend your arms alongside your legs and rest your hands beside your feet, palms facing upward. Take at least 8 deep, rhythmical breaths before progressing to the next asana.

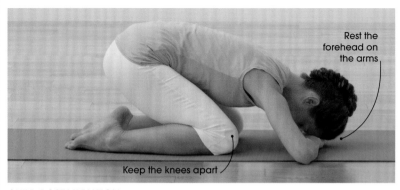

Rest the forehead on the arms
Keep the knees apart

CHILD POSE VARIATION
Sit on your heels with your knees slightly apart, lean forward, and fold your arms on the floor in front of you, hands one on top of the other. Rest your forehead on your folded arms. Take at least 8 deep, rhythmical breaths before progressing to the next asana.

"We should not confuse relaxation with laziness. In infancy the child relaxes naturally; some adults possess this power of relaxation. Such persons are noted for their endurance, strength, vigor, and vitality."

Swami Vishnudevananda

Final relaxation

At the end of every yoga session, you should practice a final relaxation lasting 15–20 minutes. This will bring about complete physical, mental, and spiritual relaxation, which is a key experience of yoga.

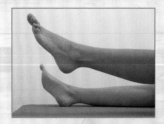

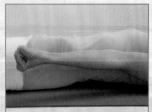

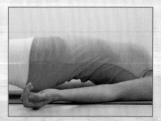

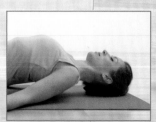

1 Inhale and lift your right leg 4 in (10 cm) off the mat. Hold your breath for a few seconds, tense your leg, then exhale and allow your leg to drop. Repeat with the left leg.

2 Inhale and lift both arms 4 in (10 cm) off the mat. Hold your breath for a few seconds, tense your arms, then exhale and allow your arms to drop to the mat.

3 Inhale and lift your hips and buttocks off the mat. Hold your breath for a few seconds, tense your buttocks, then exhale and release.

4 Inhale and lift your chest off the mat. Hold your breath for a few seconds, tense your shoulder blades, then exhale and release.

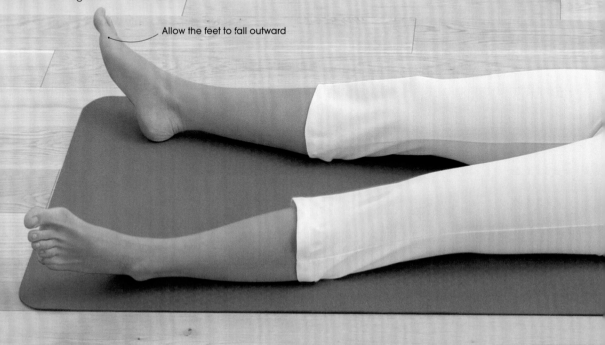

Allow the feet to fall outward

Following the sequence

Your blood pressure and body temperature will drop during final relaxation so, depending on the season, you may like to cover yourself loosely with a blanket before you begin. Follow Steps 1–8 below to achieve a comfortable Corpse Pose, then use the physical, mental, and spiritual relaxation exercises on pages 94–95 in the suggested order. Then slowly stretch and sit for a minute in a cross-legged position to end your practice with the mantra "OM."

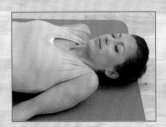 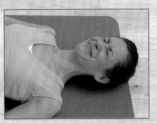 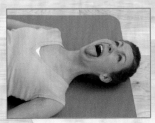 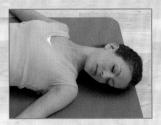

5 Inhale and pull your shoulders toward your ears. Hold your breath for a few seconds, then exhale and release your shoulders.

6 Inhale and squeeze the muscles of your face tightly together. Hold your breath for a few seconds, then exhale and release.

7 Inhale, open your mouth, stick your tongue out, and look to your forehead. Hold your breath for a few seconds, then exhale and release.

8 With an inhalation, slowly roll your head to one side; with an exhalation, roll it to the other side. End by bringing your head back to center.

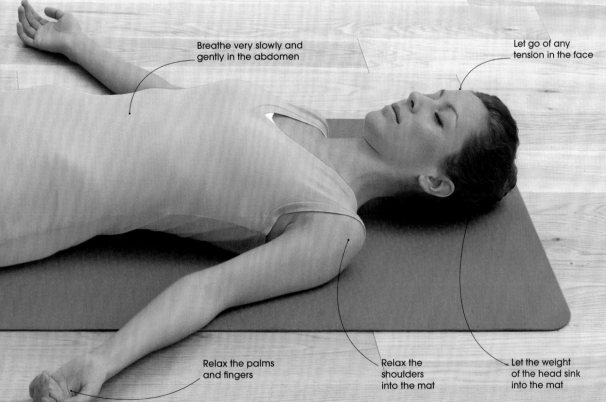

Breathe very slowly and gently in the abdomen

Let go of any tension in the face

Relax the palms and fingers

Relax the shoulders into the mat

Let the weight of the head sink into the mat

Complete yogic relaxation

Yogic relaxation has three aspects: physical relaxation, mental relaxation, and spiritual relaxation. As you lie in Corpse Pose for your final relaxation (see pp192–193), practice the thought-focusing exercises below to relax body, mind, and spirit.

Part 1: Physical relaxation

Take a few slow, rhythmic breaths using your abdomen (see p180). Then follow this exercise in autosuggestion for five to ten minutes. Have a clear mental picture of your feet, think about the downward pull of gravity, then send a mental command to your feet by silently saying, "I am relaxing my feet, I am relaxing my feet, my feet are relaxed." Move up the body; each time clearly visualize the area you are focusing on, think about the pull of gravity and your rhythmic breathing, then send a command to relax to your ankles, calves, knees and thighs, hips and buttocks, abdomen and chest, lower

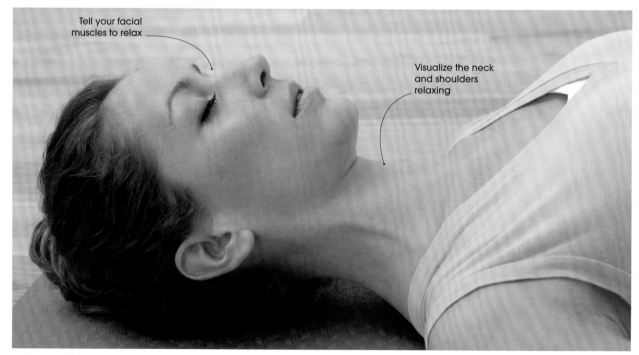

Tell your facial muscles to relax

Visualize the neck and shoulders relaxing

PHYSICAL RELAXATION

Each time you move on consciously to relax another part of the body, make sure you have a clear mental picture of that area before tuning your thoughts into the downward pull of gravity and the rhythmical flow of your breath. Finally, give the mental command to relax by silently repeating the phrase beginning "I am relaxing..."

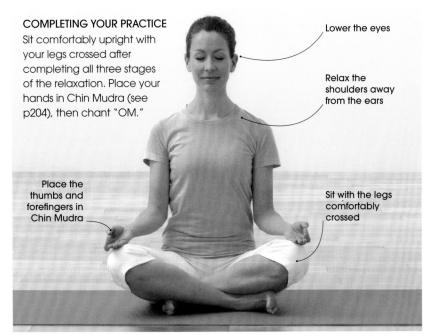

COMPLETING YOUR PRACTICE
Sit comfortably upright with your legs crossed after completing all three stages of the relaxation. Place your hands in Chin Mudra (see p204), then chant "OM."

Lower the eyes

Relax the shoulders away from the ears

Place the thumbs and forefingers in Chin Mudra

Sit with the legs comfortably crossed

> *"During spiritual relaxation the Yogi identifies himself with the all-pervading, all-powerful, all-peaceful and joyful self within himself, the real source of knowledge and strength"*
>
> Swami Vishnudevananda

back, middle back, shoulders and neck, hands and fingers, arms, mouth and eyes, facial muscles and scalp. Finally, relax your internal organs. Again, visualize the area, breathe slowly, and send the command to relax to one organ at a time: kidneys, liver, intestines, bladder, pancreas, stomach, heart, lungs, and brain. Your subconscious mind conveys the command.

Part 2: Mental relaxation

The mind is always moving between the past and the future, and in the present it is constantly pulled by the five senses. It needs to relax, so practice this mental relaxation for about two minutes. Continue abdominal breathing, this time inhaling and exhaling for five seconds each. The speed and rhythm of your breath and your thought waves are intimately linked. Start to observe the flow of air moving in and out of your nostrils. Soon your mind will be calm; if you sense it becoming active, focus on your breathing until it quiets.

Part 3: Spiritual relaxation

Complete spiritual relaxation is possible only if your thoughts have a carefree focus, so now visualize a calm lake, unruffled by waves. Picture the still water resting on your inner self, which is timeless and unchanging. Continue for five to eight minutes. Then take a few deep breaths, slowly move your legs and arms, and give your whole body a good stretch. Finally, spend a minute sitting cross-legged and chant the mantra "OM." Now you will be able to hold this sense of relaxation and focus for several hours.

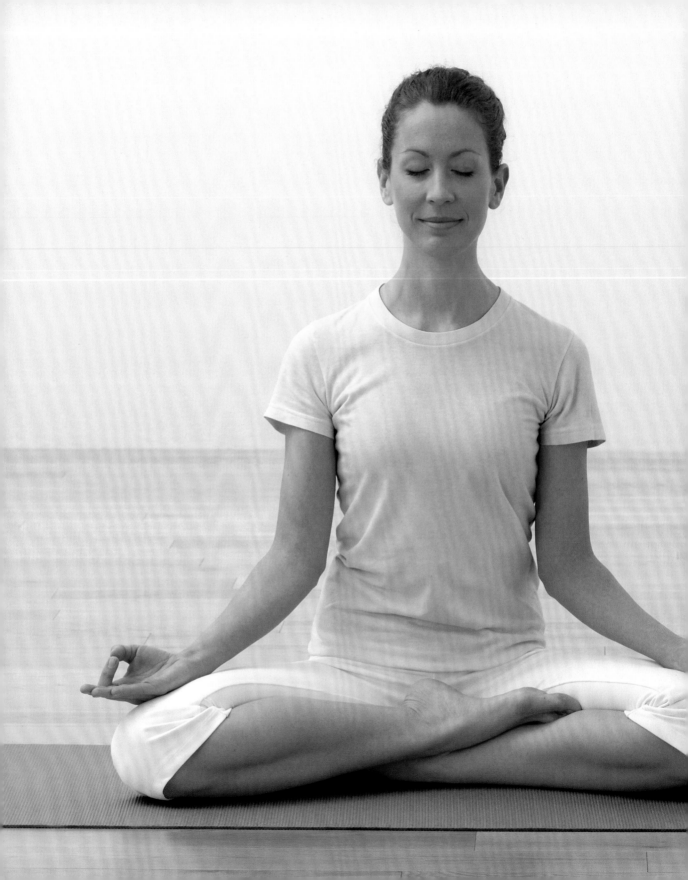

Positive Thinking and Meditation

Why meditate?

Meditation lies at the heart of any yoga practice. Once you feel comfortable practicing the asanas and breathing exercises, you will feel more relaxed in your body. Then it will seem like a natural step to pay more attention to your mind by practicing meditation. This brings about greater mental and emotional balance and, eventually, inner peace.

Physical benefits

During meditation, the distractions of the world around you disappear and the parasympathetic nervous system gently brings about a sense of relaxation and balance. Your heartbeat and respiratory rate slow and your internal organs are rested. Research shows that meditation stimulates the immune system, too, promoting health and protecting against illness.

Adepts of yoga have long recognized that the vibrations generated by thoughts and emotions affect every cell in the body—and that negative thoughts can impede the cells' capacity for regeneration and homeostasis. The focus in meditation on positive and harmonious thoughts, therefore, is thought to promote health and well-being at a cellular level.

Mental benefits

Ancient yogis aptly compared an unfocused mind to a crazy, drunken monkey, jumping from one thought to the next in a never-ending cycle. It is all but impossible to prevent the mind leaping from one thought to another. During meditation, you simply learn how to focus on the present. This prevents your mind from dwelling on the past or worrying about the future.

As your mind becomes more focused, confusion gives way to clarity. You find that you can face the conflicts that disturb your mental peace and you discover creative, positive solutions to those conflicts. This brings about a greater feeling of self-control, inner satisfaction, and sense of purpose.

What is more, you don't only experience these benefits during meditation practice. They spill over into the rest of the day, helping you to concentrate better at work and play. By encouraging emotional balance and more patience and understanding, meditation also improves your relations with those around you. You will become less irritated by other people's habits, more understanding, and better able to accept their limitations.

The ultimate goal of meditation

Ancient yogic scriptures describe the goal of meditation as *samadhi*, or cosmic consciousness.

In this state of calm understanding, the illusion of ego (the feeling that you are separate from the world) vanishes. Everything dissolves into one consciousness, or Supreme Self. In this state, you might think, "I am not my body or my mind. My mind is only my story, and I am not my story. My body does not separate me from others. I am never alone, but always one with all." All negative emotions and limiting ideas about your body and inner self vanish, setting you free from discontent. You become aware of the purpose of life and, ultimately, lose fear of death.

Experienced yogis aim to be in this state at all times, living life as one unbroken meditation. As a beginner, start by shaking free the deep-rooted habit of identifying with everything in your mind. This takes practice, but as the saying goes, every journey of a thousand miles starts with a single step.

Spiritual benefits

As your meditation practice deepens, you will gain glimpses of a state of being that you have probably never experienced before. You may feel as if life's clouds have dissipated and you can see more blue sky. You will have a sense of greater inner space, well-being, positivity, and a real feeling of trust in the goodness of life. You will start to realize that beyond the familiar world of thoughts and emotions lies a whole new realm of consciousness. Your sense of yourself will expand beyond an awareness of your body and your mind and, ultimately, you will experience a feeling of unity with everything around you.

Meditation is so powerful that its benefits extend far beyond the person who is meditating. Yogis believe that the powerful vibrations of peace that emanate from an experienced meditator have a positive effect on everyone that person comes into contact with—and that, in the end, they influence the whole world. And so making your mind peaceful through meditation is the most positive thing that you can do to contribute to world peace.

"Meditation is 'the cessation of mental activities.'" When your thoughts reduce by just 20 percent, you will experience relief and a sense of self-control."

Swami Sivananda

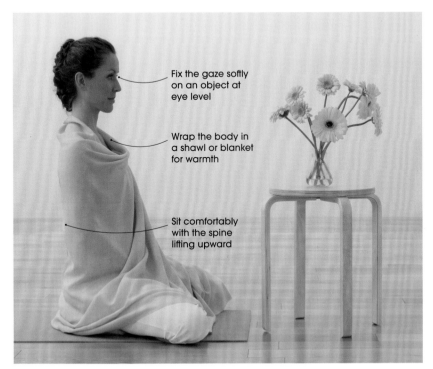

Fix the gaze softly on an object at eye level

Wrap the body in a shawl or blanket for warmth

Sit comfortably with the spine lifting upward

SITTING TO MEDITATE
When you sit to practice meditation, your physical body relaxes first. Once you feel settled, the mind begins to slow down, bringing the object of your concentration into sharper focus.

The art of concentration

Before you can learn to meditate, you have to be able to concentrate the mind. We can all concentrate to some degree, but the way we live and work today—constantly on call thanks to mobile technology and immersed in a sound-bite culture—means that many of us have only a short attention span. Practicing the simple exercises on these pages will help to lengthen your attention span and enhance your ability to concentrate, which can boost the memory and benefit your psychological health.

What is concentration?

Concentration means attending fully to one thought or object for a substantial length of time. You are concentrating when you become engrossed in a book, eat without thinking about work, or forget about your home life when in the office. The ability to concentrate is not only essential for meditation, it is key to success in any endeavor, and once you have trained yourself to concentrate effectively, you can use the skill in many other areas of life. For example, being able to shut out other thoughts and not make haphazard or hasty decisions will make you more effective at work.

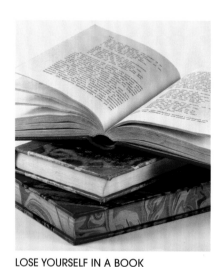

LOSE YOURSELF IN A BOOK
Read two or three pages of a book, giving them your full attention. Then test your concentration by stopping at the end of a page. How much do you remember of the story? Can you classify, group, or compare the facts you have been reading about?

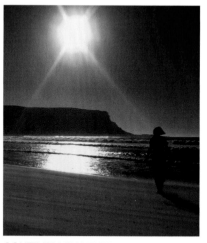

CONTEMPLATE NATURE
During the day, concentrate on the sky. Feel your mind expand as you reflect on its vast expanse. At night, concentrate on the moon or stars. By the sea, focus on waves. Or shift your gaze between objects near and far, such as a nearby tree and distant mountain.

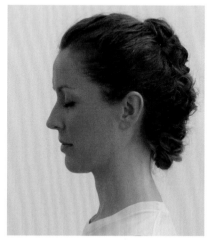

LISTEN TO A SOUND
Listen carefully to the ticking of a watch. When your mind wanders, bring it back to the sound. How long can you concentrate on that sound? Or listen to a prominent sound for a while, without reacting to it. Then shift your attention to other sounds, one by one.

The benefits of concentration

Practicing concentration has many benefits. It can strengthen "thought-currents"—how we connect thoughts and ideas in the brain—making it easier to grasp difficult, complex, or confusing concepts. It also clarifies ideas, so you can express yourself more clearly. Concentration exercises energize the mind, boosting efficiency at work and in other tasks, while building willpower and the ability to influence other people positively. They also bring about serenity, insight, and cheerfulness.

Practical exercises

The exercises below offer an easy way to develop your ability to concentrate. Initially, train your mind to concentrate on external objects, such as a book, sound, or something in nature, from waves on the ocean to stars in the sky. As you progress, you will be able to concentrate on more subtle subjects, such as an inner sound or an abstract idea. While practicing, notice how aware you are of the various qualities of the experience when the mind is focused. Then note how difficult it is to assimilate an experience with an unfocused mind. When your mind wanders—which it will do often—remind it to come back to contemplation of the object or quality you are focusing on. Gradually lengthen your practice until you can concentrate for half an hour.

"Emotional balance maintained in all activities is the true sign of progress ..."

Swami Sivananda

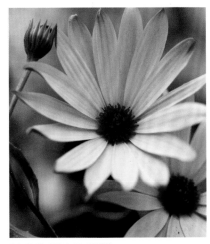

FOCUS ON A FLOWER
Sit comfortably with your eyes closed. Imagine a garden with many flowers. Gradually, bring your attention to a single flower. Visualize its color and explore its other qualities, such as texture, shape, and scent. Concentrate on the flower's qualities for as long as possible.

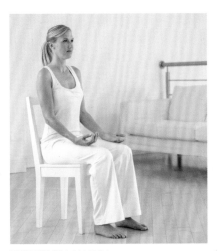

REFLECT ON AN IDEA
Relax your body and mind and think about a quality, such as compassion. Imagine how you could express it in your life. Think of great people who embodied it. Ask the quality to fill your heart, then to flow out to the whole world. Think of yourself as perfectly compassionate.

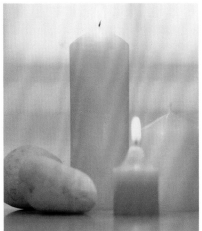

CANDLE CONTEMPLATION
Sit cross-legged in a dark room with a lit candle at eye-level an arm's distance away. Watch your breath for 2–3 minutes. Then look at the flame for 1 minute. Try not to blink. Close your eyes and visualize the flame between your eyebrows for a minute.

Practicing meditation

Meditation is a state of relaxed awareness. Swami Vishnudevananda used to say that it is not possible to teach someone how to achieve this state, any more than it is possible to teach someone how to sleep. However, the more care and attention you give to your preparation for meditation, the more positive the results will be. This preparation can be divided into two parts: first become comfortable with physical meditation, then focus your mind with mental meditation (see p204).

Physical meditation

If you get the atmosphere right for meditation, the purity of the space will be so tangible that at times of stress you can sit in your meditation space, practice for half an hour, and experience great comfort and relief.

PLACE It's best to set aside a special room for meditation, but if this is not possible, try to separate one portion of a room to use for your practice. Keep it clean and tidy, and make a focal point by placing a candle and a spiritually uplifting picture at eye level in front of the place you sit for meditation. Gazing at the steady candle flame before starting a meditation practice helps to concentrate your mind and turn it inward. Burning incense can also help to create a meditative mood. You will need a clean mat or folded woollen blanket to sit on. Many yogis like to place it to face north or east to take advantage of favorable magnetic vibrations. With repeated practice, the vibrations created during meditation will build a magnetic aura. Within six months, the peace and purity of the atmosphere should be tangible.

TIME The best times for meditation are at dawn and dusk, when the atmosphere is thought to be charged with a special spiritual force. At dawn, in the quiet hours after sleep, the mind is especially clear and unruffled. If this hour is tricky, practice at dusk or just before going to bed. Alternatively, find a time when you are free from daily activities and your mind can be calm.

HABIT Practice every day at the same time. As your subconscious mind gets accustomed to the regularity, you will find it easier to settle and focus. Start with 15 to 20 minutes, building up to one hour (aim for at least 30 minutes). It is better to meditate every day for 30 minutes than once a week for two hours.

"Feel the silence, hear the silence, touch and taste the silence. Silence is the music of your soul."

Swami Vishnudevananda

SITTING POSITION Sit on the floor to meditate, in a position that you can maintain comfortably, keeping your spine and neck straight but not tense. You do not have to sit in the classic Lotus posture—a simple, cross-legged pose makes a firm base, or you can sit in Half-lotus pose (see below). Sitting on a cushion helps the thighs to relax and brings the knees closer to the ground. In all these sitting positions, the legs make a triangular pattern. This shape contains the energy raised during meditation rather than allowing it to disperse in all directions.

If you can't sit on the floor easily, sit on a comfortable chair with your ankles crossed. Do not lie down to meditate—you will relax too completely and may fall asleep. Choose one of the three hand positions shown on p204.

BREATHING Once you are sitting comfortably, relax your body as much as possible, especially the muscles of the face, neck, and shoulders. Broaden your chest and lift your rib cage to encourage Abdominal Breathing, which brings oxygen to the brain. Then inhale and exhale rhythmically for about 3 seconds each, slowing your breath to an imperceptible rate. Notice how your breath becomes lighter and completely silent.

Sitting positions

Whichever position you choose, make sure it is comfortable—you should be able to sit with a straight spine without fidgeting for up to 30 minutes. If you find these poses too stressful on your hips or knees, sit on a chair. Then choose a hand position (see p204).

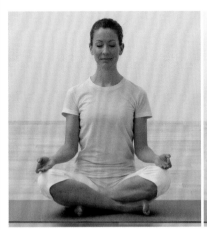

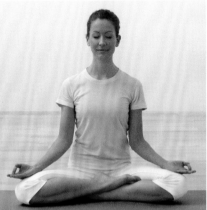

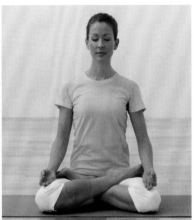

CROSS-LEGGED POSE
Sit comfortably upright and bend your knees, crossing one shin in front of the other. Try to relax your knees toward the floor.

HALF-LOTUS POSE
Sit comfortably with your legs wide and bend one knee, bringing the sole against your groin. Place the opposite foot on top of the bent leg.

LOTUS POSE
Sit with crossed legs. Raise your front leg and place the top of the foot on the opposite thigh. Carefully lift the other foot onto the other thigh.

Hand positions

Once you are sitting comfortably, lift your spine and relax your shoulders. Rest your hands in one of these hand gestures, or *mudras*, to keep the arms and shoulders relaxed and to focus your prana, or vital energy.

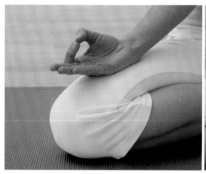

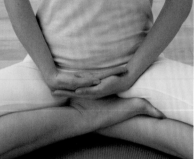

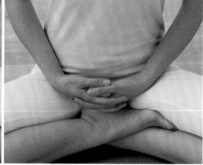

CHIN MUDRA
Rest the backs of your palms on your knees or thighs and join the tips of your thumbs and forefingers. Extend the other fingers.

CUPPED HANDS
Turn both palms to face upward in front of your groin and gently cup the back of your right hand in your left palm.

CLASPED HANDS
Turn both palms to face upward in front of your groin and interlink your fingers, resting one thumb on top of the other.

Mental meditation

Follow these meditation techniques to stabilize your mental energy and to focus your mind. But first, simply allow your mind to wander. If, initially, you are too eager to control your mind, you might develop a headache.

GIVE THE MIND SPACE Focus deeply on your breathing to give your mind space. Then watch your mind closely. Be patient and compassionate with it: developing a trusting relationship with your mind ensures its cooperation.

DISASSOCIATE If your mind wanders, watch it objectively, as if watching a film. Just observe your thoughts for a few minutes and they will diminish.

CONCENTRATION POINT Bring your awareness to a chakra (see p179). If you relate easily to others, focus on the heart center (anahata chakra) at the center of your chest. If you are analytical, focus on the self-awareness center (ajna chakra), between your eyebrows. Aim to keep this focus for life.

CONCENTRATION OBJECT Focus on a symbol; try something concrete, such as the sun or sky, or a positive quality, like love or kindness. Or try a mantra, such as "OM." Repeat the sound mentally, in time with your breath.

"During meditation, we watch our mind without expectation. Sustained attention combined with detachment ultimately unveils the ocean of wisdom that lies within"

Swami Vishnudevananda

Managing stress

It is now widely acknowledged, even by mainstream medicine, that meditation is very useful for treating depression and stress-related conditions. To understand how this works, it is helpful to know about the physiological changes that occur when we are feeling stressed, known as the "fight or flight response." This programming helped ancient man to deal with emergencies requiring a huge amount of physical effort, such as fighting off an animal.

The body's stress response

The "fight or flight response" activates the nervous system, and chemicals are released into the bloodstream, among them adrenaline, noradrenaline, and cortisol. These increase your rate of breathing, dilate your pupils to sharpen your eyesight, and direct blood away from your digestive system toward your muscles, readying the body for physical effort. Thanks to these changes, your reflexes quicken, you feel less pain, and your immune system gets ready for action. You suddenly perceive everything as a threat to survival, and are quick to react with anger or aggression and less likely to behave positively. We once needed such responses to ward off physical danger, but today, most stress is psychological, caused by work or relationships. And where in the past stress was resolved by fighting or running away, it now may not have a clear end. If the nervous system does not get a message that danger has passed, the "fight or flight response" persists; over time, this causes burnout.

COMBATING STRESS For your body to function well again, you must activate the parasympathetic nervous system. You can do this by following the physical preparation for meditation (see pp202–203), sitting quietly and breathing rhythmically. Then use the mental preparation techniques (see opposite) to relax your mind, focus it on a positive goal, and distance it from the stressor. You might also like to use positive affirmations to view your situation in a new light. Try saying, "I allow myself to relax. I am alive and I can breathe. This situation is temporary and will end. Help is available." Then focus your mind on a peaceful natural scene, a harmonious sound, or a pleasant memory. Or visualize a sage or saint, and feel powerful, soothing vibrations entering your heart. This creates a calm sense of connection with something greater than yourself, giving you confidence to deal with the causes of stress.

Stress-busting tools

Start dealing with symptoms of stress as soon as you notice them using these simple strategies.

Counter shallow breathing by taking a few deep abdominal breaths. Use your diaphragm fully and make the exhalations long.

Sit comfortably on a chair with your back straight, feet on the floor, palms on your thighs, and your eyes closed. Breathing deeply, bring your attention to areas of your body in which you feel tension. Ask each part to relax. Repeat three times with full attention and confidence.

If you work long hours at a computer, practice eye exercises two to three times a day and regularly look at the sky through a window.

If you sit for most of the day, get up every hour and do some stretches. Bend forward for a few seconds, then bend backward. Twist to the right, then to the left. Finally, stretch sideways.

The law of karma

In yoga, the purpose of meditation is linked to the law of karma—the belief that everything happens for a reason and that every action has a reaction. Your meditation practice will guide your mind toward the positive thinking that will attract joy into your life. Swami Sivananda advised people to focus on a single positive quality for a whole month—the chart opposite will help you to do just that.

What is karma?

The law of action and reaction teaches that doing good deeds attracts goodness to us and, conversely, that doing bad deeds attracts ill. This is true of thoughts as well as deeds. The reaction provoked by a thought will be of the same nature and quality as the thought itself, so a negative thought attracts a negative reaction and a positive thought a positive one. Today, we tend to believe that others are responsible for what happens to us, especially for the more challenging episodes. We are quick to blame parents, teachers, or society at large for our ills. We fail to realize that our negative thoughts and emotions—fear of failure, resentment, anger, self-hatred—generate powerful, negative vibrations. These attract negative energy that influences events, the people we meet, and even the diseases we get. For example, dwelling on unhappy memories and worrying that painful things will happen again sets up a vibration of fear, which attracts fear and pain. This is the law of karma.

BEING RESPONSIBLE FOR YOUR LIFE Understanding the law of karma brings the realization that you are responsible for your own life. It is no use blaming others or outside events for the ills you suffer. The secret of happiness and pain rests in your hands—or, rather, in your mind. If the universe brings you only and exactly those things that are on the same wavelength as your thoughts and feelings, the key to happiness is to pay attention to what you think and feel. You are the architect of your own destiny. So if you find yourself thinking a negative thought, try quickly to correct it with a more positive one.

A HABIT OF POSITIVE THINKING Whenever possible, think joyous, happy, and harmonious thoughts. Yogis believe that these bring well-being to mind and body. Practicing meditation is a good way to guide your mind toward the positive; if you practice in the early morning, the effects remain with you all day. Or you could repeat the positive affirmation of the day (see opposite.)

"Yogis insist that the mind can and should be very dynamic and that it is the quality of our inner world that determines the quality of our lives."

Swami Sivadasananda

A year of positive thinking

Start each day by concentrating on the quality of the month, shown below. Allow its energy to vibrate in your mind and visualize the benefits of interacting with others using this quality. Repeat once during the day, then end your day with a short meditation on that thought. By the end of a month, you will have developed a habit of positive thinking.

January	February	March	April
Patience	**Compassion**	**Adaptability**	**Cheerfulness**
"I trust that life will bring me what I need."	*"I have compassion for all beings."*	*"I adapt easily to new circumstances."*	*"I meet each situation with a cheerful mind."*

May	June	July	August
Love	**Peace**	**Courage**	**Will**
"I intend to greet each person with love."	*"My mind remains peaceful in all circumstances."*	*"I am full of courage."*	*"My will is all-powerful."*

September	October	November	December
Humility	**Detachment**	**Self-confidence**	**Endurance**
"I surrender to the cosmic will."	*"I look at my life circumstances from a new perspective."*	*"I trust that my inner self is pure positivity."*	*"I regard all difficulties as opportunities to grow."*

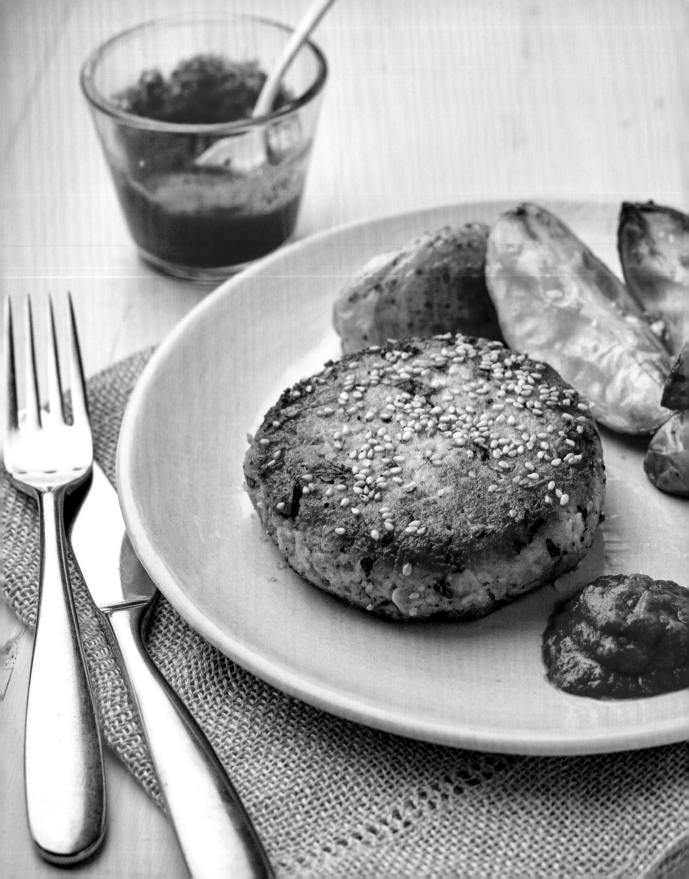

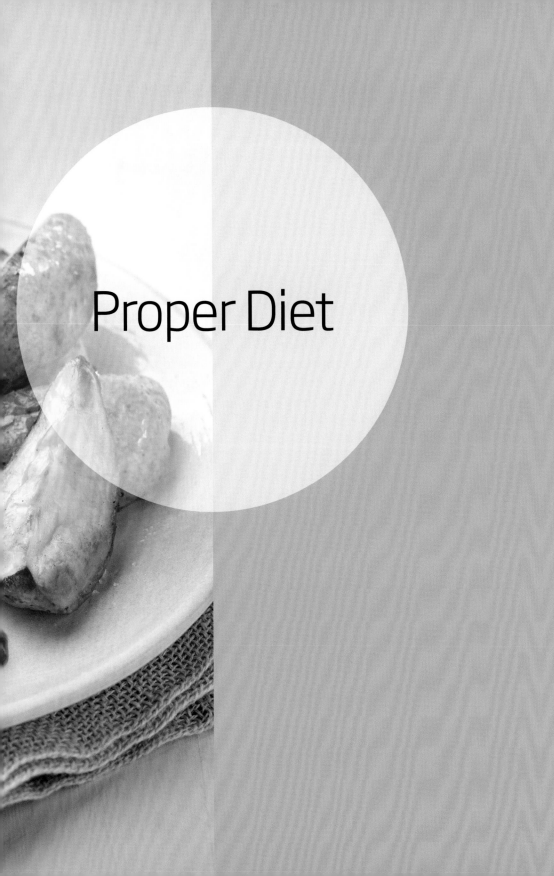

Proper Diet

Yoga and vegetarianism

The yogic tradition advocates a lacto-vegetarian diet—avoiding meat, fish, and eggs, and limiting your dairy intake. Predominantly plant-based, this diet ensures that your food gets its energy directly from the sun, the source of all life. Your food should also be freshly prepared and, ideally, organic.

Why be a vegetarian?

According to yogic tradition, a non-vegetarian diet violates the principle of ahimsa, the sanctity of all living things. But there are also many health benefits to vegetarianism. Research shows that vegetarians living in affluent countries enjoy remarkably good health and live longer than their meat-eating counterparts. They are slimmer, have lower blood pressure, and suffer less from heart disease, diabetes, dementia, and many cancers.

THE PROBLEM WITH MEAT Meat contains large amounts of cholesterol, saturated fat, and potentially carcinogenic (cancer-forming) compounds, including pesticide residues. When meat is grilled or fried, it forms carcinogenic polycyclic aromatic hydrocarbons, while cured and smoked meats contain nitrates and nitrites that may increase the risk of cancer, particularly among children. The findings of the China Study in 2006 indicated that the lower the percentage of animal-based foods in the diet, the greater the health benefits, and that getting one's nutrients from plant-based foods actually reduced the development of cancerous tumors.

Another concern about meat is that crowded factory farms are fertile breeding grounds for salmonella, e.coli, listeria, and campylobacter. What is more, the hormones, antibiotics, and vaccines that are given to animals leave residues that are believed to pose a threat to human health.

THE BENEFITS OF PLANT FOODS Plant foods contain dramatically higher amounts of antioxidants, fiber, and vitamins. They also contain a host of phytonutrients that appear to offer protection against many cancers, assist in hormone balance, protect the heart, and help reduce blood pressure.

Following a vegetarian diet also offers a way of living an environmentally conscious lifestyle. Just think of this: it takes 2,500 gallons (11,000 liters) of water to produce 1lb (500g) of meat, but only 25 gallons (110 liters) to produce 1lb (500g) wheat. It's easy to see why many argue that the most efficient way to feed the world's population is with a vegetarian diet.

Getting Your Calcium

Calcium is essential for bone health and to ensure efficient muscle contraction and blood clotting. If you are following a lacto-vegetarian diet, you have a number of options for getting enough calcium in your diet.

Everyone needs to eat 6–8 servings daily of foods that are rich in calcium. Below are some examples of foods that will give you one serving of a calcium-rich food:

- 4¼oz (120g) cooked quinoa

- 4oz (115g) cooked or 8oz (230g) raw broccoli, kale, bok choy, okra, or spinach

- 1fl oz (30ml) tahini

- 4fl oz (125ml) cow's milk, yogurt, or fortified soy milk

- 6oz (130g) dried apricots or currants

THE LACTO-VEGETARIAN FOOD PYRAMID

This vegetarian food pyramid is based on the latest research and reflects the total daily nutritional needs of an average adult woman. If you lead an active lifestyle, exercising regularly 2–3 times a week, you will need to increase your intake of all food groups. If you are older or less active, you will need to decrease your intake.

The foundation of the pyramid is whole grains—the mainstay of a healthy vegetarian diet. The average adult woman should eat 6 servings daily. Next come pulses, dairy, nuts, and seeds—aim for 5 servings daily. The next largest intake is vegetables—aim for 4 servings daily. These are the most important source of vitamins, minerals, and phytonutrients. Next comes fruit—aim for 2 servings daily. Finally, eat fats and oils sparingly—not more than 2 servings daily.

Fats and oils

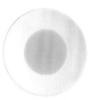

Olive oil
2 servings, any vegetable oil = ½fl oz/ 2 tsp (10ml)

AN EASY MEASURE FOR SERVINGS

The cup measurements are an easy way to measure ingredients. You can also use a liquid measuring cup in the same way, as follows:

1 cup = 8 fl oz (230ml)
½ cup = 4 fl oz (115ml)
¼ cup = 2 fl oz (55ml)

Fruit

Apples
1 serving, raw = 3oz (90g)

Berries
1 serving, any soft fruit = 3oz/½ cup (75g)

Vegetables

Red peppers
1 serving, raw = 3oz/1 cup (90g)

Broccoli
1 serving, raw = 3oz/1 cup (90g)

Salad leaves
1 serving, any green salad = 1¼oz/1 cup (35g)

Pumpkin
1 serving, raw = 5oz/1 cup (140g)

Pulses, dairy, nuts and seeds

Tofu
1 serving = 4oz/½ cup (110g)

Flageolet beans
1 serving, any pulses, cooked = 3oz/1 cup (90g)

Nuts & seeds
1 serving, any = 1½oz/¼ cup (40g)

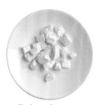

Feta cheese
1 serving, any soft cheese = 1oz/¼ cup (30g)

Chickpeas
1 serving, any pulses, cooked = 3oz/1 cup (90g)

Wholegrains

Whole wheat bread
1 serving = 1 thin slice 1¼oz (35g)

Whole wheat pasta
1 serving, cooked = 2½oz/½ cup (70g).

Quinoa
1 serving, cooked = 3½oz/½ cup (95g)

Bulgur wheat
1 serving, cooked = 3oz/1 cup (90g)

Granola
1 serving = 2½oz/½ cup (75g)

Brown rice
1 serving, cooked = 3½oz/½ cup (100g)

You are what you eat

According to the Upanishads, the ancient scriptures of India, food is Brahman—the Divine reality. When we eat we are unified with the environment and with each other. Our food produces the energy that drives our body, but it also shapes our emotions and affects our minds.

Eating with awareness

We live in an age where fast is considered better, and many of us eat hurried meals. Eating in a hurry means that you do not have time to really taste what you are eating, to know when you have eaten enough to satisfy hunger, or to notice the effect that a certain food has on your mood or emotions. On a physical level, hurried eating impairs digestion. On an emotional and psychological level, it separates us from the food we eat. The yogic way is to eat mindfully, being aware of what you are eating and where you are eating it.

ATTITUDE TO FOOD Adopt a balanced, joyful approach to what you eat. Enjoy it, respect it, and be grateful for it. It is a gift of nature. When you cook, your emotions are transferred to the food. Always prepare food with love, allowing your prana to pass to the food and nourish the people you are feeding.

HOW TO EAT Make sure that you are comfortable when you are eating. Always sit down and eat somewhere peaceful. If you eat alone, be silent. If you are with friends or family, avoid arguments and emotional issues. Eat slowly so you really taste the food, chew your food well to prepare it for the stomach, and do not overeat. Keep your awareness on the act of eating.

WHEN TO EAT Eat three meals at regular times each day and always wait until your last meal is digested before eating again. Do not eat if you are not hungry and do not eat a large meal late at night. At bedtime, avoid heavier foods such as dairy and pulses.

WHAT TO EAT Eat unrefined, organic food, preferably locally produced and in season. Do not eat fruit with meals as it may cause bloating and indigestion. Try and eat the lighter food in a meal first. Only sip a little warm water at mealtimes. Liquids dilute the digestive enzymes and impair digestion. Never drink ice-cold water at any time as it is too cold for the body.

The gunas

Sattva This is the quality of purity, truth, light, and love; the higher quality that allows spiritual growth. Sattvic foods promote physical, mental, and spiritual health and they calm the mind. They are fresh, pure, and full of prana. They are also easy to digest and free from chemicals, pesticides, fertilizers, and preservatives. Sattvic foods should make up most of your diet.

Rajas This is the quality of change, activity, and movement. Rajasic foods are stimulating by nature; they include warmed-up or overcooked foods, as well as stale or rotten foods. Used in moderation, they provide the body with vital energy, but in excess, they create imbalance, which leads to restlessness, hyperactivity, and anger.

Tamas This is the quality of dullness, darkness, and inertia. Tamasic foods lead to sluggishness, dullness, and lethargy, and incline the body toward disease. They are difficult to digest and are lacking in prana. Tamasic foods are the ones to be most avoided. They include food that is old, stale, or reheated; leftovers; microwaved food; and canned and frozen food.

Types of food

In the yogic way of eating it is important to keep the three gunas (sattva, rajas, and tamas) in balance. Food is categorized according to the effect it has on each of the gunas. The need to balance the gunas explains why certain foods are not permitted in a yogic diet, even if, to the Western way of thinking, they do not have detrimental physical effects.

	Sattvic foods	Rajasic foods	Tamasic foods
Grains	Freshly prepared grains: rice, whole wheat, oatmeal, barley, millet, unleavened bread	Very hot or salty grain-based foods, e.g. salted porridge; fried bread	Foods made from refined flour: white pasta, pizza, commercial breakfast cereals
Vegetables	Most fresh vegetables and salads	Onions, leeks, radishes, garlic, okra, potatoes, carrots, karela, peppers, chili peppers	Mushrooms
Fruit	Most fresh fruit and freshly made juices; fresh dates are considered highly sattvic	Unripe fruit, lemons, limes, olives, avocado, tomatoes, bottled juices	Canned and sweetened, fermented, and frozen fruit
Sweet foods	Honey; raw, unrefined sugar	White sugar (for its short-term effects), malt syrup, corn syrup, mollasses	White sugar (for its long-term effects), pastries, chocolate, ice cream, jams
Seasoning	Mild spices: cumin, coriander, fennel, fenugreek, cardamom, cinnamon, saffron	Vinegar; hot spices, e.g. chili, cayenne; mustard; pickles; strong herbs; salt; soy sauce	Pickles and relishes
Pulses	Freshly prepared pulses, e.g. mung beans, aduki beans, black and brown lentils	Very hot or salted pulses	Canned or frozen pulses
Proteins	Nuts (especially almonds); sesame seeds; sunflower seeds; tofu; fresh, pure milk	Eggs, hard cheeses, peanuts, salted nuts, sour cream	Meat; fish; salted nuts; texturized soy protein; milk, pasteurized or homogenized
Drinks	Pure, fresh fruit juice; fresh milk; fresh lassi; herbal teas	Coffee, tea, small amounts of alcohol	Alcohol; soft drinks; milk, pasteurized or homogenized
Fats	Fresh, organic unsalted butter, ghee, and yogurt; olive oil; sesame oil; flax oil	Salted butter, fried fruits	Deep-fried food, lard, margarine

Common concerns about the yogic diet

If you have never tried a vegetarian diet, you are bound to have a lot of questions about it. And if you are a yoga practitioner, or thinking of starting yoga, you may want to understand more about how vegetarianism can support you in your yoga practice.

"Why does the yogic lacto-vegetarian diet include milk and cheese when research shows that these are linked to health problems?"

Traditionally, milk, cream, butter, and yogurt are Sattvic foods (see pp212–213) and favored in a yogic diet. However, with modern dairy farming methods, the degree to which you include dairy in your diet is a matter of personal choice. Cow's milk contains residues of antibiotics and hormones that have been shown to disrupt hormone levels in men and women. Pasteurization and homogenization destroy milk's beneficial bacteria, which makes milk hard to digest and contributes to the rise in dairy allergies and digestive problems.

But the body needs fat; butter and fresh cheese are a good source of nutrients and are not harmful in small amounts. Also, a little dairy can help practically and emotionally if you are trying to switch to a totally vegan diet.

"I practice yoga for at least two hours each day. How will I be able to get enough protein to maintain and build my muscles and strength on a yogic lacto-vegetarian diet?"

It is a myth that you need high levels of protein in order to exercise. Some of the strongest and biggest animals on earth eat a plant-based diet. The "protein myth" stems from some poor experiments in the 1900s on the protein requirements of rats. Human protein requirements, measured in experiments the 1950s, indicated that most complex carbohydrates (like those in beans, grains, and vegetables) have all the amino acids required by humans.

Moreover, the once commonly held belief that vegetarians need to eat specific combinations of plant proteins in the same meal to achieve "complete proteins" has been dispelled. We now know that the body has a pool of stored amino acids to complement the amino acids in recently digested food.

In addition, your protein requirements are probably lower than you think. According to the World Health Organization, protein only needs to be five percent of our total calorie intake. Virtually every single lentil, bean, vegetable, nut, seed, grain, and fruit provides more than five percent of its calories as protein, and some have much higher levels.

Nor is protein an efficient source of energy. Muscle fatigue sets in when carbohydrate stores in the muscles and liver are depleted, so diets that are high in carbohydrates (found in whole grains, vegetables, and pulses) will prevent fatigue and muscle damage. If you exercise to a particularly strenuous level, then a protein-rich meal or snack, such as sunflower seed butter on whole grain toast, after your exercise, will help to prevent depletion of the amino acids in your body.

What this means is that, as long as you are eating enough calories to meet your energy requirements, and not eating a diet full of junk and refined food, then the lacto-vegetarian diet can easily meet all your protein needs.

"I've heard about the acid-alkaline balance. What does this mean and does it have anything to do with vegetarianism?"

Acid is produced in our body for a number of different reasons and generally speaking, the acid-alkaline levels are very precisely controlled by complex biochemical mechanisms. The metabolism of our food and our lifestyle choices can produce a great deal of acid. Whenever we exercise, or even move, our body produces acid. When we get stressed, our acid levels rise. Foods such as animal products, refined grains, fats, and sugar are acid-forming, as are alcohol, coffee, black tea, peanuts, walnuts, preservatives, and hard cheeses.

Too much acid in the body leads to acidosis, which is when acid is deposited in our tissues. This can lead to a multitude of diseases—gout, rheumatism, gall and kidney stones, arteriosclerosis, and heart disease. Migraines and cancers have also been linked to high levels of acidity. And it gets worse. To counteract high levels of acid, the body may take alkaline salts, such as calcium, from the bones. This can lead to osteoporosis.

To combat acidosis, do your yoga practice. Yoga is renowned for being a stress-busting tool. In addition, you should aim for 80 percent of your food and drink to be alkaline-forming. This is where being a vegetarian comes in. Most plant foods, with the exception of lentils, are alkaline, and even if you eat lentils a few times a week, providing you are following an organic vegetarian diet, then the lentils should not cause you any problems.

"Can diet help my powers of concentration for yoga?"

It is recommended that you follow a Sattvic diet. If your diet is too Rajasic (see pp212–213), you will be restless and unable to sit in meditation. If it is Tamasic (see pp212–213), you will feel too heavy and dull to think with clarity. Avoid stimulants such as tea, coffee, and chocolate.

In addition, we know that the neurons in the brain need essential fats to function properly, so include a small amount of seeds and nuts, and their oils, in your diet. Flax and hemp are particularly good. Finally, use rosemary and sage in your cooking or to make infusions. Rosemary is a cerebral stimulant, while sage can clear emotional obstructions from the mind and promote calmness and clarity.

The transition toward a yogic diet

This six-week plan will help you to work toward either a lacto-vegetarian or a vegetarian diet. For best results, make the changes gradually and adjust the diet to your own needs. Be aware that

Week 1

- Start to take meals at regular times. Eat slowly and chew your food well.
- Check your pantry and use up, donate, or give away processed foods such as white sugar, cookies, and canned sauces.
- Shop for organic products only, including in-season fruit and vegetables; whole grains and pulses; cold-pressed oils for cooking and salad dressings; meat, fish, eggs, and dairy foods.
- Reduce meat portions and use more vegetables. Cut out processed meats such as sausages, salami, and burgers.
- Cut out all soft drinks such as colas and artificially-sweetened juice drinks.

Tip of the week

"Make one vegetarian dish. Read the recipes in this book for ideas."

Week 2

- Stop eating all red meat. Replace beef, lamb, and pork with lighter meats such as fish or chicken.
- This week, make two vegetarian main meals. Use chickpeas, lentils, and adzuki beans instead of meat in lasagne or casseroles. Try cooking with tofu.
- Try different whole grains with each meal, including brown rice, quinoa, and couscous. Chew them well to avoid bloating and wind.
- Try alternatives to coffee made from cereal grains, or reduce the number of cups you drink.
- Have three alcohol-free days this week. Try fresh juices diluted with sparkling water.

Tip of the week

"Visit a bookstore and choose an inspiring vegetarian cookbook."

Week 3

- If you feel ready, cut out all meat. If you miss the texture of meat, use thick slices of eggplant or nut loaves.
- Reduce all your portion sizes of fish and eggs, and increase your portions of vegetables.
- Restrict your intake of tea or coffee to no more than two cups a day.
- Continue to cut back on your alcohol intake.
- If you are eating out, try some vegetarian options. Most restaurants offer a good choice.
- Focus on chewing each mouthful 5 to 10 times more than you usually would; also, keep each sip of liquid in your mouth for about 10 seconds, gently swirling it around. This will gradually make you "eat your drink and drink your food," helping you be more satisfied by your meals and have better digestion, too.

Tip of the week

"Try a vegetarian dish if you are eating out, most restaurants offer a good choice."

you may experience some symptoms of detoxification, like headache, fatigue, or skin problems. If this happens, slow down. You may need six months or longer to achieve your goal.

Week 4

• Don't eat fish more often than every other day. Use the menu planner (see pp220–221) to plan for three fish-free days.

• If you miss eating more traditional meat dishes, look online or in cookbooks for vegetarian versions of your favourite recipes. Try the Veggie-tofu burgers on page 228.

• Reduce tea and coffee to one cup per day.

• Don't feel guilty if you haven't reached all your goals. Look at what you are finding most difficult and work out how to make things easier.

Tip of the week

"Invite friends for dinner and cook them a vegetarian meal."

Week 5

• Reduce your fish intake to two days this week.

• If you eat eggs every day, try to cut down to every other day.

• Try using egg alternatives, such as a banana for each egg in cakes or pancakes, or buy egg replacers from your local health food store.

• If you feel your meals are too light, add a little cold-pressed flaxseed or olive oil to dress your vegetables, or make a tahini dressing (see p230). Make sure you are eating enough whole grains.

• See if you can avoid alcohol completely, except on special occasions.

• If family or friends ask you for dinner, let them know that you would prefer not to eat meat or fish–but don't push your ideals upon them.

Tip of the week

"Tell family and friends that you are working toward a healthier diet."

Week 6

• Stop eating all fish and eggs, and enjoy a wide variety of plant foods.

• Make sure that you are eating the correct number of servings of all the food groups (see the food pyramid p211).

• Expand your repertoire of recipes by searching in cookbooks or on the internet.

• Don't give yourself a strict time limit for changing your diet. Instead of worrying about what you haven't yet achieved, feel proud of the things you have managed to do.

Tip of the week

"Congratulations! You've made the change to a healthy yogic diet."

Cooking techniques

Grains and legumes are key to a lacto-vegetarian diet, but people often find them hard to digest. It is important to know how to cook them properly to avoid bloating, gas, or indigestion. Washing and soaking before cooking removes dirt and makes them more digestible. Oils are used in a lacto-vegetarian diet to replace animal fats. Knowing how to store oils correctly to prevent them from turning rancid is important.

Grains

The key to cooking grains is to measure or weigh them so you know how much water to use. The table below shows you the correct proportion of grains to liquid to produce a yield of 3½ cups of cooked grains.

SOAKING AND RINSING Most grains, except for quinoa and millet, will be more digestible if you soak them in cold water before cooking for at least 30 minutes or preferably overnight. Quinoa and millet may be dry-roasted for a few minutes instead. Whether or not you have soaked them first, before cooking rinse the grains in cold water 2–3 times, ideally until the water runs clear.

COOKING Bring the correct amount of water to a boil (see chart), add the grain, and a pinch of salt. Bring back to a boil, reduce the heat, and cover. Simmer until the water has been absorbed. Remove from the heat but leave for a few minutes in the covered pan before serving to dry out the grains.

Cooking times and water volumes

Grain	1 cup grain	Volume of water	Cooking time	Yield (cups)
Barley	7oz (205g)	2½ times	35–40 minutes	3½
Buckwheat	5¾oz (170g)	2–2½ times	35–40 minutes	3½
Bulgur wheat	6oz (175g)	2 times	35–40 minutes	3½
Couscous	6½oz (185g)	2 times	15 minutes	3½
Millet	6¾oz (195g)	3 times	25–30 minutes	3½
Oats, rolled	4oz (115g)	2¾ times	10 minutes	3½
Quinoa	6½oz (180g)	2 times	15–20 minutes	3½
Rice, white basmati	7oz (205g)	2 times	15–20 minutes	3½
Rice, brown basmati	7oz (205g)	2½ times	30–35 minutes	3½
Rice flakes	3½oz (105g)	1¼ times	5–7 minutes	3½
Wild rice	6½oz (180g)	4 times	50 minutes	3½

Legumes

Many people have problems digesting beans and pulses. They can cause flatulence and allergies. If you are just starting to add beans to your diet, eat them no more than 1-2 times a week for the first few weeks. After that you may be able to increase your consumption to 3-4 times per week. The most easily digested beans are split mung beans, aduki (adzuki), and black gram beans, sometimes known as urad dal. Following the guidelines below will make beans easier to digest:

SOAKING AND RINSING Always soak beans before cooking. This helps remove the oligosaccharides (a form of carbohydrate) that cause flatulence. Soak for 4 hours or overnight in 3-4 times their volume of water. Soak fava beans and older beans for 24 hours. Rinse before cooking.

COOKING Cook in fresh water. You may need as much as 6 times their volume of water as some of the water evaporates during cooking. Bring to a boil, partially cover, and simmer until soft. Never eat undercooked beans and do not boil them or add salt or acid ingredients, such as large amounts of lemon juice or tomatoes. This can make them tough and hard to digest.

SERVING Adding ginger, fennel, cumin, or black pepper to cooked beans aids digestion. Traditionally, these spices are sautéed in ghee or oil, then added to the finished dish.

Oils

Research shows that trans fats contribute more than unsaturated fats to cardiovascular disease. Trans fats are formed when oils are exposed to heat and air, so it is vital to know how to store oils and which to use for cooking.

STORING Always store oils in a dark place and choose oils that are packaged in dark glass or metal containers. Avoid those that are sold in clear plastic bottles. Stable oils—such as ghee and olive oil—can be stored in a dark cupboard. Cold pressed oils, such as avocado, flaxseed, safflower, and sunflower oils are very unstable and should be kept in the fridge.

COOKING For cooking at high temperatures, especially above 320°F (160°C/Gas 3), as when baking in the oven, only use the most stable oils. Choose from organic ghee, organic sesame oil, palm kernel oil, or coconut oil. You can sauté food at moderate temperatures using olive oil. Never use the unstable, cold-pressed oils mentioned above for cooking.

A week's menu

The week's menu plan given below will help to ease your transition to a vegetarian diet. For each day of the week there is a suggested breakfast, lunch, and dinner, as well as some snacks and

	Monday	Tuesday	Wednesday
Breakfast	• Vanilla milk rice with almonds *p224*	• Breakfast smoothie *p224*	• Apple cinnamon oatmeal *p222*
Lunch	• Couscous with mozzarella and arugula *p227* • Digestive lassi *p249*	• Pasta with green pesto *p233* • Salad greens with orange tahini dressing *p230*	• Mung dal soup *p226*, served with steamed brown basmati rice • Endive with yogurt dill dressing *p231*
Dinner	• Upma *p232* • Pink raita *p231*	• Vegetable soup with ginger *p235* • Parathas *p240*	• Bulgur wheat with roasted zucchini sticks *p233* • Pink raita *p231*
Snacks and sweet treats	• Chocolate muffins *p244*	• Fresh organic fruit with mixed seeds	• Open rice-paper wraps *p246*

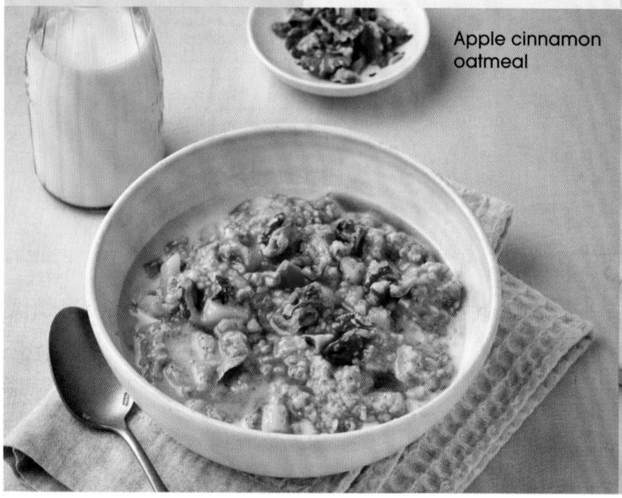

Apple cinnamon oatmeal

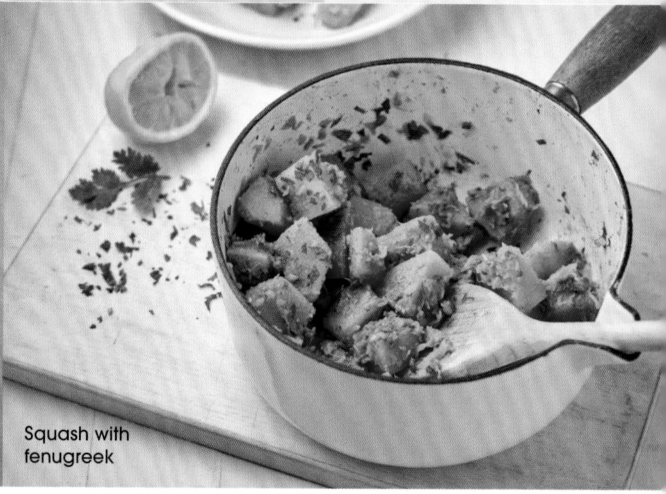

Squash with fenugreek

sweet treats. All the recipes are found in this chapter. The plan has been designed for variety and interest, but you should feel free to make substitutions to suit your own taste.

Thursday	Friday	Saturday	Sunday
• Veggie tahini spread *p225*, served with toasted rye bread	• Apple cinnamon oatmeal *p222*	• Vanilla milk rice with almonds *p224*	• Chocolate delight *p225*, served with toasted whole wheat bread • Fresh organic fruit salad
• Rajma *p227* served with simple boiled quinoa • Coconut chutney *p239*	• Mung dal soup *p226*, served with boiled brown rice or bulgur wheat • Squash with fenugreek *p236*	• Cillas *p241* • Date and fig chutney *p239* • Vegetable soup with ginger *p235*	• Tofu veggie burgers *p228* • Baked potato wedges *p238* • Yogic ketchup *p238* • Lemonade with fresh mint and orange-blossom water *p249*
• Pasta with green pesto *p233* • Green beans with pine nuts *p238*	• Upma *p232* • Mint and cilantro chutney *p239*	• Bulgur wheat with roasted zucchini sticks *p233* • Guacamole *p248*	• Parathas *p240* • Broccoli with toasted almonds and lime seasoning *p236* • Coconut chutney *p239*
• Vegetable sticks with goat's cream cheese dip *p248*	• Very simple oatmeal spice cake *p244*	• Vanilla pears with a creamy filling *p242*	• Cardamom-ginger Highland shortbread *p245*

Cillas served with chutneys

Vegetable soup with ginger served with Parathas

Breakfast

In our fast-paced world, breakfast all too often consists of a snatched coffee and croissant or a processed high-sugar cereal. Instead, start your day as you mean to go on: take at least 15 minutes to eat slowly and in a relaxed environment, enjoying freshly prepared whole grains that will sustain your mood and energy.

Apple cinnamon oatmeal

Oats are an excellent source of fiber and nutrients because they are naturally rich in bran, germ, and protein. The apple adds the key vitamins and the cinnamon lends a delicious hint of spice.

Serves 4

2 sweet apples

4½oz (125g) rolled oats,
or buckwheat or millet flakes

pinch of salt

2 tsp ground cinnamon

4 tbsp chopped walnuts, or other
nut of choice

4 tbsp maple syrup, or agave
syrup, honey, raw cane sugar,
or crumbled jaggery

14fl oz (400ml) milk of choice, such
as cow's, rice, almond, or soy

1. Peel, core, and dice the apples (leave them unpeeled if they are organic).

2. In a saucepan, bring 1¾ pints (1 liter) water to a boil. Add the oats, apples, salt, and cinnamon. Cook over a low heat for about 10 minutes, stirring frequently with a whisk.

3. Heat a frying pan over medium heat. Add the nuts and toast for about 5 minutes, or until they become fragrant and darken slightly.

4. Divide the oatmeal between four serving bowls. Add maple syrup or sweetener of choice and a splash of milk. Sprinkle the toasted nuts over the top and serve.

Notes

- Never add uncooked fresh fruit to your oatmeal as the combination of fresh fruit and grains is hard to digest.

- If you choose honey as sweetener, let your oatmeal cool down to 104°F (40°C) before you add it. Honey loses its natural beneficial properties if too hot!

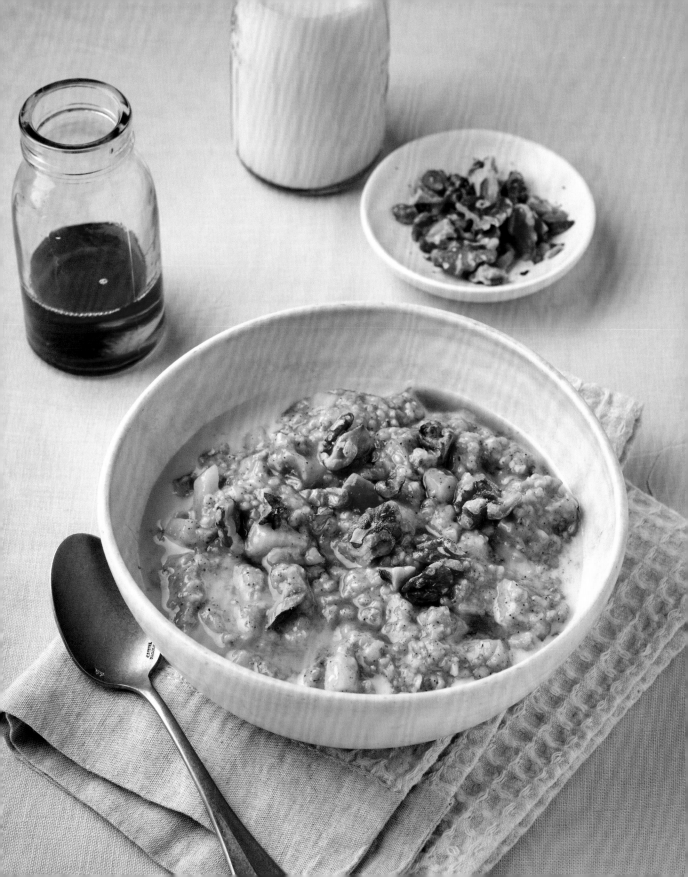

Vanilla milk rice with almonds

Creamy and satisfying, this makes a lovely nutritious breakfast with a
hint of sweet spice. It also makes an excellent dessert.

Serves 4

12 whole almonds, skins on, soaked
in cold water overnight

6 dried dates, pitted

7oz (200g) broken white rice, such
as basmati or jasmine

½ vanilla pod (split), or 1 tsp
powdered vanilla (see note)

1 pint (600ml) milk of choice, such
as cow's, rice, almond, or soy

4 tsp coconut oil, or ghee or butter

1 tsp ground cardamom

4 tbsp light raw cane sugar,
or agave syrup

1. Drain the almonds, then remove skins and halve. Chop
the dates into small pieces. Set almonds and dates aside.

2. Bring the rice and 1 pint (600ml) water to a boil in a medium
saucepan. Add the vanilla pod, cover, turn heat to low, and cook
for about 10 minutes, until the rice is soft. Stir vigorously with a
wooden spoon until the rice takes on a creamy, sticky texture.

3. Add the milk, almonds, and dates, and mix well. Cook
over a low heat for a further 5 minutes, stirring continuously.

4. Remove from the heat and add the coconut oil,
cardamom, and sugar or agave syrup. Mix well and serve.

Notes

- If using powdered vanilla, it will give more flavor if added at the
  end with the sweetener, coconut oil, and cardamom.
- Unbroken rice can be used, but cook for an extra 10 minutes.

Breakfast smoothie

This crunchy, revitalizing drink will help boost your brainpower and
concentration. Almonds and cashews are rich in essential minerals, while
dried figs and dates are crammed with antioxidants and also add a
delicious natural sweetness.

Serves 4

2½oz (75g) whole almonds, skins on

2½oz (75g) cashew nuts

16 dried dates, pitted

8 dried figs

1 pint (600ml) water (more if you
prefer a less thick smoothie)

pinch of saffron

½ tsp ground cardamom

2 tbsp rosewater

1. Soak the almonds, cashew nuts, dates, and figs overnight
in cold water, using a separate bowl for each. Next day, drain,
discarding the soaking water from the nuts, but reserving the
water from the dried fruit.

2. Soak the saffron for a few minutes in a little warm water.
Remove the skin from the almonds.

3. Place soaked nuts and fruit in a blender or food processor,
along with the soaking water from the dried fruit and the rest
of the ingredients. Blitz until your smoothie is creamy but still
slightly crunchy, and serve.

Chocolate delight

This fabulous spread keeps well in the fridge for up to four days.

Serves 4

5 tbsp ground almonds or hazelnuts

4½oz (125g) unsalted butter at room temperature, or margarine or coconut oil

5 dried figs, finely chopped

10 dried dates, pitted and finely chopped

4 tbsp honey, or agave or maple syrup

2½ tbsp cocoa powder

1 tsp ground cinnamon

1. Heat a frying pan over medium heat. Add the ground almonds or hazelnuts and toast until they are fragrant and darken slightly. Transfer to a mixing bowl and leave to cool.

2. When the toasted nuts are cool, add the remaining ingredients to the bowl. Stir until well combined. Serve spread on whole wheat toast.

Note

- This also makes a great cake filling or topping.

Veggie tahini spread

Tahini makes this spread a rich source of health-boosting vitamins and minerals.

Serves 4

1 carrot, peeled and grated

½ fennel bulb, peeled and grated

⅛ celeriac root, peeled and grated

4 tbsp tahini

1 tsp salt

pinch of freshly ground black pepper

4 tbsp finely chopped fresh green herbs, such as sage, basil, rosemary, or dill

2 tsp lemon juice

1. Place the carrot, fennel, and celeriac in a bowl.

2. Add the tahini and season with the salt and pepper.

Stir together, then add the chopped herbs and lemon juice. Gently stir again to combine all of the ingredients. Serve spread on whole wheat toast.

Note

- You can transform this spread into a delicious pasta sauce by adding some hot water and extra seasoning and herbs to taste.

Lunch

Lunch is the key meal of the day. Even if you have a busy work schedule and little time to spare, it should still be possible to include at least one cooked grain, one cooked vegetable, and, depending on the season, a small serving of raw vegetables in the form of a salad. Extra protein can be provided by including tofu or beans, a small serving of soft cheese, or a sprinkling of nuts or seeds.

Mung dal soup

This is the yogi's standard lunch because, when paired with brown rice, it contains all the essentials of a balanced vegetarian diet. The mung beans provide energy-giving proteins, the vegetable curry adds the vital vitamins, and the rice offers wholesome yet easy to digest carbs.

Serves 4

For the dal

5¾ oz (160g) dried split mung beans

½ large cinnamon stick, or ½ tsp ground cinnamon

6 cardamom pods, lightly crushed, or ½ tsp ground cardamom

2 tsp turmeric

2 tsp salt

7oz (200g) fresh spinach leaves, or the green part of Swiss chard, washed and torn

2 tsp lemon juice

1 sprig of fresh coriander, to garnish

For the curry base

4 tsp olive oil, or sesame oil or ghee

1 tsp whole cumin seeds

2 tbsp fresh root ginger, peeled and finely chopped

⅛ fresh green chili, or pinch of chili powder

1 tsp ground cumin

2 tsp ground coriander

¼ tsp ground cloves

½ tsp ground nutmeg

1. Rinse the mung beans in a sieve under cool running water. Place in a large saucepan with 1½ pints (900ml) water. If using the cinnamon stick and cardamom pods, add these to the pan as well. If using ground cinnamon and cardamom, add these to the curry base in step 3. Stir in the turmeric.

2. Bring to a boil. Skim off any white foam that appears on the surface using a slotted spoon. Reduce the heat and let simmer for 30 minutes. Add the salt and the spinach or Swiss chard, then leave to simmer for a further 10 minutes.

3. Meanwhile, prepare the curry base. Heat the oil or ghee in a small pan. Add the cumin seeds, ginger, and chili, then stir in all the ground spices, including the ground cinnamon and ground cardamom, if not using whole spices in step 1. Once the spices give off a fragrant aroma (this will only take a few seconds), remove the pan from the heat and stir in 3 tablespoons water. The pan will still be hot enough for the water to evaporate, leaving a paste or curry base. Be careful this does not burn or it will spoil the taste of the soup.

4. Stir the curry base into the dal, along with the lemon juice. Garnish with fresh coriander leaves and serve.

Couscous with mozzarella and arugula

Here is a creative way to enjoy a freshly prepared hot lunch at your workplace. All you need is an electric kettle and a heatproof bowl with a lid.

Serves 4

7oz (200g) couscous

1 tsp salt

pinch of freshly ground black pepper

small handful of arugula, washed and torn

7oz (200g) mozzarella cheese, or smoked tofu, diced

12 black olives, pitted

4 tbsp olive oil

juice of ¼ lemon

1. Put the couscous, salt, and pepper into a heat-resistant bowl. Pour over 15fl oz (450ml) freshly boiled water, cover, and leave to stand for 10 minutes.

2. Gently fold the arugula, mozzarella or tofu, and the olives into the couscous. Drizzle the olive oil and lemon juice over the top.

Rajma

This hearty casserole-style meal is rich in protein. Contrary to their reputation, legumes can be eaten without causing flatulence–the secret lies in cooking them long enough and using the proper spices.

Serves 4

5½oz (150g) dried red kidney beans, soaked overnight in cold water

4 firm, ripe tomatoes

4 tbsp cooking oil of choice

1 tsp black mustard seeds

2 tsp whole cumin seeds

2 tsp fresh root ginger, peeled and finely chopped

12 curry leaves

1 tsp ground cumin

2 tsp ground turmeric

pinch of chili powder

1 tsp ground coriander

2 tsp curry powder

½ tsp ground cinnamon

2 tsp salt (or more according to taste)

8 potatoes, peeled and diced

4 carrots, peeled and diced

2 zucchini, diced

4 celery sticks, diced

2 tbsp finely chopped fresh coriander, to garnish

¼ lemon, sliced, to garnish

1. Drain and rinse the kidney beans. Place in a large pan with plenty of fresh water, bring to a boil and cook for about 1 hour, or until tender. Drain and set aside.

2. Put the tomatoes into a bowl of just-boiled water for 2–3 minutes. Remove from the water using a slotted spoon and, when cool enough to handle, peel off the skin, then coarsely chop.

3. Heat the oil in a wok or large saucepan over high heat. Add the mustard seeds. When they start to pop, add the cumin seeds, then after a few seconds add the ginger and the curry leaves. Fry for 30 seconds, then stir in the ground cumin, turmeric, chili powder, ground coriander, curry powder, cinnamon, and salt.

4. Add the chopped tomatoes to the wok and stir-fry for 3 minutes. Then, add the potatoes along with 8fl oz (250ml) hot water. Turn heat to low, cover with a lid, and cook for 10 minutes. Add the carrots, zucchini, and celery. Cover again and cook until the vegetables are tender—about 10 to 15 minutes.

5. Stir in the kidney beans and cook for another 2–3 minutes, until heated through, adding extra hot water if you prefer your curry more soupy. Serve garnished with fresh coriander and lemon slices.

Tofu veggie burgers

This is the perfect meal to make your kids happy or to gently introduce confirmed carnivores to an alternative way of eating. Any leftover burgers are delicious eaten cold with a dab of the Yogic ketchup.

Serves 4

8oz (225g) celeriac, peeled

1 medium fennel bulb, stems trimmed

2 medium carrots, peeled

14oz (400g) firm tofu

1 bunch fresh parsley or basil

4 tbsp rice flour, or chickpea flour or cornflour

3 tsp salt

½ tsp coarse ground black pepper

2 tsp ground nutmeg

4 tbsp brown sesame seeds

4 tbsp cooking oil of choice

Yogic ketchup (see page 238), to serve

Baked potato wedges (see page 238), to serve

1. Finely grate the celeriac, fennel, and carrots. Rinse the tofu under cold running water, pat dry, and then also finely grate.

2. Remove and discard any hard stems from the parsley or basil, then finely chop.

3. Combine the grated vegetables, tofu, flour, parsley or basil, salt, pepper, and nutmeg in a large bowl, until well combined. Using your hands, shape into 8 small, flat burgers about ¾in (2cm) thick, pressing them firmly so they hold together—you may need to use more rice flour to help them bind. Set aside in the fridge for about 30 minutes to allow the burgers to firm up.

4. Remove from the fridge and sprinkle each side of the burgers with the sesame seeds. Gently press the sesame seeds into the surface of the burgers so they stick.

5. Heat the oil in a non-stick frying pan over medium heat. Fry the burgers for about 5–7 minutes on each side, until they are crispy on the outside, but still soft inside. Serve with Yogic ketchup and Baked potato wedges on the side.

Tofu veggie burgers served with Yogic ketchup and Baked potato wedges – both recipes on page 238.

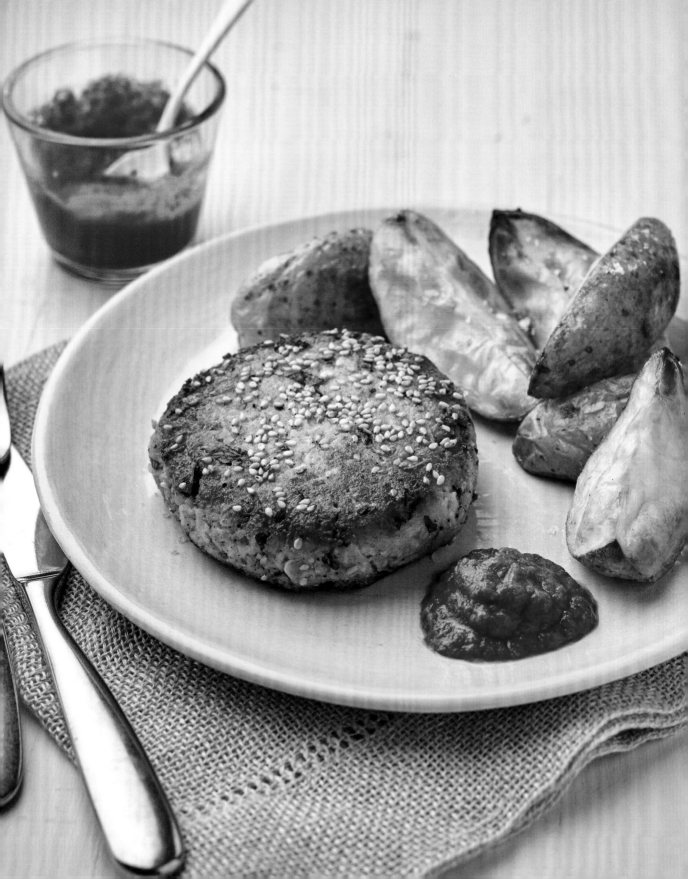

Salads and dressings

Raw foods are an important source of prana (see p178) and enzymes. Salads are a great way to include raw vegetables, leaves, and herbs in meals, but because they are hard to digest they are best eaten as a side dish at lunchtime, when digestion is at its strongest.

Salad greens with orange tahini dressing

This salad comes with a lovely dressing that does not require any salt and is rich in vitamin C. It also makes a great sauce for steamed vegetables.

Serves 4

For the salad

½ Bibb lettuce, or other salad leaves of choice, such as Batavia, oak leaf, Romaine, or baby spinach

½ cucumber, peeled and sliced

2 firm, ripe tomatoes, washed and sliced, or 8 cherry tomatoes, halved

4 tbsp alfalfa sprouts, rinsed and drained (optional)

For the dressing

10fl oz (300ml) freshly squeezed orange juice

4 tbsp lemon juice

6 tbsp thick tahini

1. Mix the lettuce, cucumber, tomatoes, and alfalfa sprouts in a salad bowl.

2. Prepare the dressing by using a blender to mix the orange juice, lemon juice, and tahini together to form a creamy sauce. Let the dressing sit for 5 minutes to allow it to thicken. If it is too thick, add a little more orange juice; if it is too runny, add a little more tahini.

3. Drizzle the dressing over the salad and serve.

Endive with yogurt dill dressing

Here crisp endive is combined with a dressing that is both low in fat and rich in taste.

Serves 4

4 small endives

7oz (200g) yogurt, full or low fat

4 tbsp lemon juice

small handful fresh dill, finely chopped, plus 1 sprig to garnish

salt

pinch of ground black pepper

1. Wash and drain the endive and tear it into single leaves. Arrange the leaves on a salad platter or on 4 salad plates.

2. Prepare the dressing by whisking the yogurt, lemon juice, dill, salt, and pepper into a creamy dressing.

3. Pour the dressing over the endive, garnish with a sprig of dill, and serve.

Note

• Vegans can use soy or coconut yogurt.

Pink raita

Raita is really a dip and can accompany almost any hot Indian-style meal, for example Upma (see p232) or Bulgur wheat with roasted zucchini sticks (see p233). If you eat it regularly, prepare a larger quantity and keep in an airtight container in a cool, dark place.

Serves 4

2 tbsp cumin seeds

2 beets, peeled and finely grated

7oz (200g) yogurt

pinch of chili powder

salt

small handful of fresh coriander or flat-leaf parsley, finely chopped

1. Toast the cumin seeds in a dry frying pan over medium heat until they turn fragrant and darken slightly—be careful not to burn them! Allow to cool, then grind to powder, using a pestle and mortar or an electric coffee grinder.

2. Put the grated beets into a bowl, stir in the yogurt, cumin, chili powder, salt, and half of the fresh coriander or parsley. Garnish with the remaining coriander or parsley and serve.

Notes

• As a shortcut, you can use store-bought ground cumin, but don't toast it!

• You can lightly steam the beets before use.

• Vegans can use soy or coconut yogurt.

Dinner

According to yoga and the science of ayurveda, the evening meal should be light and easy to digest, as our digestive capacity is not as strong at night and our metabolism slows. As a result, a heavy, late evening meal may place a burden on your liver, leading to the formation of toxins, or *ama*. Eat three hours before bedtime and avoid dairy products and big servings of pulses—soups, pastas, and stews are good options. Try these recipes and see if you wake up in the morning with more energy for the day ahead.

Upma

Originally from South India, this dish is now popular all over the subcontinent. The recipe is quick and very easy to make and is also highly nutritious.

Serves 4

6oz (175g) semolina
4 tbsp oil or ghee
1 tsp black mustard seeds
2 tsp cumin seeds
1 tsp fenugreek seeds
2 tsp urid dal (optional)
4 tbsp raw cashew nuts
¼ tsp finely chopped green chili, or a pinch of chili powder
2 tsp fresh ginger, finely chopped
12 curry leaves (optional)
2 tsp salt
2 carrots, peeled and finely chopped
5½oz (150g) green peas, or finely chopped green beans
2 tbsp lemon juice
fresh coriander sprigs, to garnish

1. Heat a dry frying pan over high heat. Add the semolina to the pan and toast it for about 5 minutes, until it becomes fragrant and turns golden brown. Remove from heat and set aside.

2. Heat the oil or ghee in a medium saucepan or large frying pan, add the mustard seeds and cook them until they start to pop. Now add the cumin seeds and fenugreek seeds, urid dal (if using), and the cashew nuts and fry for 2–3 minutes until they all start to brown. Now add the chili, ginger, curry leaves (if using), salt, carrots, and green peas or green beans. Fry for a minute, then add 16fl oz (500ml) water and bring the mixture to a boil.

3. Stir in the toasted semolina, and cook over low heat for 5 minutes, stirring constantly. The upma should be a crumbly texture when done, but if it looks too dry, add some more water. Serve, sprinkled with the lemon juice and garnished with coriander sprigs.

Notes

- Use chopped fresh coriander instead of curry leaves, if you wish.
- For a gluten-free alternative, substitute polenta or rice flakes for the semolina. If using rice flakes, soak them for 5 minutes in warm water instead of toasting, and do not add more water after adding them to the vegetables.

Pasta with green pesto

The pesto keeps fresh in the fridge for up to two days. Besides serving with pasta, it is also delicious with simple boiled potatoes.

Serves 4

5½ oz (150g) raw cashew nuts or almonds, peeled

4 tbsp pine nuts

scant 1oz (25g) mixed fresh green herbs such as basil, sage, and rosemary

pinch of salt

4 tbsp olive oil

½ tsp ground black pepper

4 tsp lemon juice

8 tbsp grated Parmesan or pecorino cheese (optional)

11oz (325g) whole wheat pasta

1. Heat a dry frying pan over high heat. Add the cashew nuts and pine nuts and toast until they turn golden brown and are fragrant. Leave to cool.

2. Make the pesto by putting the toasted nuts, green herbs, salt to taste, olive oil, and black pepper in a blender or food processor. Blend together, gradually adding enough water to form a thick, creamy sauce. Blend in the lemon juice and, if you are using cheese, blend half of it into the pesto.

3. Cook the pasta in plenty of boiling salted water until al dente. Drain and stir the pesto through it.

4. Serve immediately, sprinkled with the remaining grated cheese.

Note

- You can use gluten-free pasta instead of whole wheat.
- Vegans can omit the grated cheese from the pesto.

Bulgur wheat with roasted zucchini sticks

A combination of boiled, light grains and gently cooked zucchini makes an excellent dinner. It is nutritious enough not go to bed feeling hungry, but digestible enough to allow for a restful sleep.

Serves 4

7oz (200g) bulgur wheat

½ tsp salt, plus more to taste

4 tbsp olive oil

3 zucchini, washed and cut into large sticks

freshly ground black pepper

4 tbsp sunflower seeds

2 tsp lemon juice

4 tbsp finely chopped fresh mint

1. Put the bulgur wheat into a large saucepan, add 15fl oz (450ml) water and ½ tsp salt, cover with a lid and bring to a boil. Once the water starts to boil, reduce the heat and let it simmer for 10 minutes without stirring or lifting the lid.

2. Meanwhile, heat the oil in a frying pan over medium heat. Add the zucchini sticks, cover the pan, and cook, keeping the lid on and turning the zucchini occasionally, until they are tender—about 12 minutes. Remove from the heat, add salt and pepper to taste, sprinkle with the sunflower seeds, lemon juice, and mint, and serve with the cooked bulgur wheat.

Notes

- Chutney is a tasty a addition to this dish.
- If you prefer, you can bake the zucchini in the oven at 400°F (200°C/Gas 6) instead of frying them.
- For a gluten-free option, quinoa can be substituted for the bulgur wheat. Cook for 20 minutes.

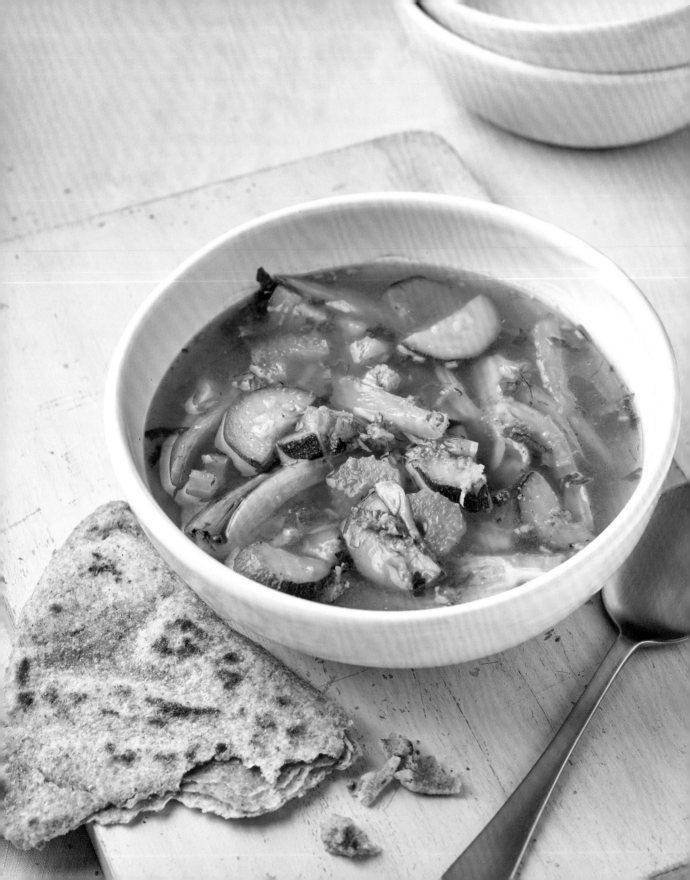

Vegetable soup with ginger

A warming, light soup is easy to digest and ideal for dinner as it will not overload the stomach before going to sleep. To make into a more substantial meal, add cubed potatoes to your vegetable mixture or serve with freshly made Parathas (see p240).

Serves 4

4 tbsp olive oil

4 tbsp fresh ginger, finely chopped

2 zucchini, trimmed and cut into half-moon pieces

2 fennel bulbs, trimmed and cut into quarters

4 celery sticks, trimmed and cut into 1¼in (3cm) pieces

4 tsp salt

4 tsp curry powder

1¾ pints (1 liter) water

1 tsp ground nutmeg

4 tsp lemon juice

4 tbsp shredded fresh coriander, to garnish

1. Heat the oil in a large pan over medium heat. Add the ginger and fry for about 30 seconds. Add the vegetables, salt, curry powder, and nutmeg, and stir-fry for another 5 minutes.

2. Add the water to the pan. Bring to a boil, cover, and cook over a low heat for 8 minutes.

3. Turn off the heat. Stir in the lemon juice and serve, garnished with the shredded fresh coriander.

Notes

- Fresh parsley or basil also make an excellent garnish for this soup.
- You can use a mixture of almost any vegetables. Try using colorful alternatives such as kale, carrots, or white beets. Use a total weight of around 14oz (400g) of vegetables.

Vegetable soup with ginger served with Parathas (see p240).

Vegetables and condiments

Vegetables are not only an excellent source of vitamins and minerals, but also contain phytonutrients that are thought to protect against cancer. They have an alkalizing effect on the body, so should form a large part of everyone's diet. In addition to the vegetables in your main dish, always try to include some cooked vegetables as a side dish.

Broccoli with toasted almonds and lime seasoning

Rich in antioxidants and vitamin C, broccoli is one of the most powerful foods to support the immune system. It also helps build strong bones and body tissue.

Serves 4

4 tbsp whole almonds, skinned and halved

1¾lbs (800g) broccoli, washed and cut into florets, with stems peeled and sliced

2 tbsp lime or lemon juice

4 tbsp sesame oil

salt and freshly ground black pepper

1 tsp ground nutmeg

2 tbsp finely chopped fresh mint

1. Toast the almonds in a hot, dry frying pan until they turn golden brown. Transfer to a small plate to cool down.

2. Cook the broccoli by steaming for 3-4 minutes or boiling in very little water for 6–8 minutes, until cooked but still firm.

3. Prepare the seasoning by mixing together the lime or lemon juice, oil, salt and pepper to taste, and nutmeg using a whisk or fork. Stir in the chopped mint and drizzle the seasoning over the cooked broccoli. Sprinkle toasted almonds on top, and serve.

Squash with fenugreek

In this recipe, starchy squash is balanced out with bitter fenugreek seeds and tangy lemon juice. Rich in fiber and antioxidants, fenugreek seeds are helpful in keeping the digestive system in good health by flushing out toxins.

Serves 4

4 tsp ghee, sunflower oil, or sesame oil

2 tsp fenugreek seeds

1 tsp ground turmeric

2 tsp salt

1 pinch chili powder

1 large Hokkaido or butternut squash, peeled, deseeded, and diced

4 tbsp lemon juice, plus lemon wedges to garnish

1 large bunch of fresh coriander, finely chopped, reserving sprigs to garnish

1. Heat the ghee or oil in a large pan over medium heat. Add the fenugreek seeds, then after 15 seconds add the turmeric, salt, and chili powder. Add the diced squash and stir-fry for 5 minutes. Cover the pan and leave to cook for 15–20 minutes, stirring occasionally, until the squash is tender.

2. Remove the pan from the heat and gently fold in the lemon juice and the finely chopped coriander. Garnish with lemon wedges and sprigs of fresh coriander.

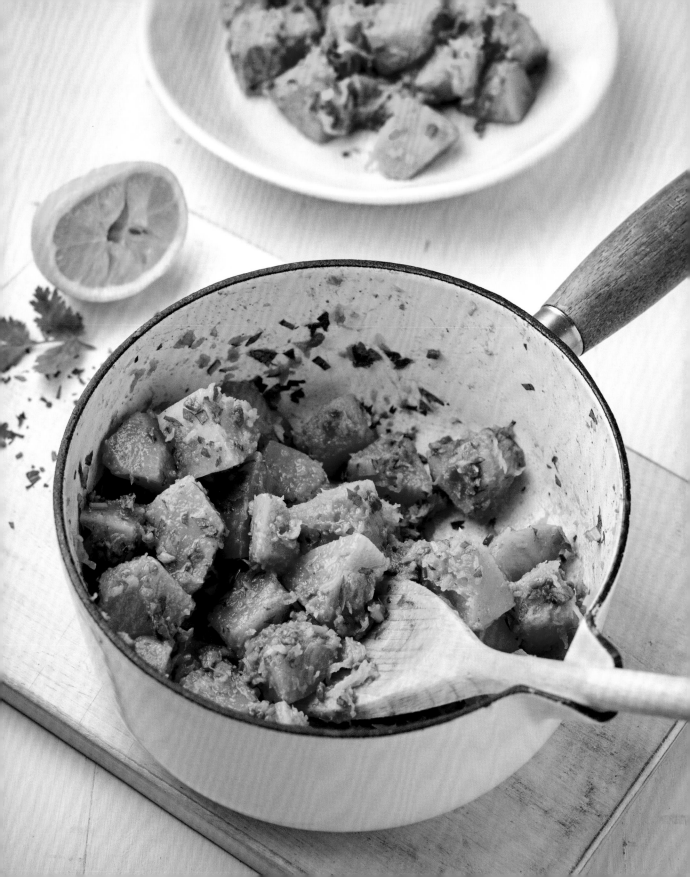

Green beans with pine nuts

Green beans have a high fiber content and are a rich source of vitamins A, C, and K. Pine nuts contain a good amount of magnesium and anti-aging antioxidants and add the delicious Mediterranean touch to this simple dish.

Serves 4

4 tbsp pine nuts

4 tbsp olive oil

1¾lb (800g) green beans, trimmed

salt and freshly ground black pepper

4 tbsp finely chopped fresh sage

2 tbsp lemon juice

4 tbsp crumbled goat's cheese, or feta cheese

1. Heat a dry frying pan over high heat. Add the pine nuts and toast until they turn golden brown. Remove pan from the heat and transfer the pine nuts to a small plate to cool.

2. Heat 1 tbsp olive oil in a saucepan, add the green beans, salt and pepper to taste, and 4 tbsp water. Cover, bring to a boil, and cook over low heat until the beans are tender—about 20 minutes, adding more water if needed. For the last 30 seconds, add the sage.

3. Remove from the heat, drain off any water, and stir in the lemon juice and remaining olive oil. Transfer to a serving dish, sprinkle the crumbled goat's cheese and the toasted pine nuts on top, and serve immediately.

Notes

- Fresh rosemary can be substituted for the sage.
- Smoked tofu can be substituted for the goat's cheese to make this dish vegan-friendly.

Baked potato wedges

Great on their own, especially when served with Yogic ketchup (see below), these are the perfect match for the Tofu veggie burgers on page 228.

Serves 4

12 medium-size potatoes, peeled (leave unpeeled if organic) and quartered lengthways into wedges

4 tbsp olive oil

salt

1. Preheat the oven to 400°F (200°C/Gas 6).

2. Place potato wedges in a bowl with the olive oil. Toss so wedges are well coated in the oil. Place on a baking tray and sprinkle with salt to taste.

3. Bake in the hot oven for 40 minutes, or until the wedges are crisp on the outside and tender inside.

Yogic ketchup

This is a vast improvement on the store-bought variety. It will keep well for up to 3 days in the fridge.

Serves 4

4 firm, ripe , medium tomatoes, cored and diced

4 sundried tomatoes, diced

2 tsp olive oil

4 tsp tamari

2 tsp ground paprika

pinch of chili powder

4 tsp lemon juice

4 tsp maple syrup

1. Put the fresh and sundried tomatoes, olive oil, and 4 tbsp water in a blender or food processor and blitz to form a thin puree, adding more water if necessary.

2. Place the puree in a saucepan. Add the tamari, paprika, and chili powder, and bring gently to a boil. Cover and leave to simmer over a low heat for about 25 minutes, adding more water if the mixture starts to become too dry.

3. Remove from the heat and stir in the lemon juice and maple syrup. Transfer the ketchup to a bowl and leave to cool down.

Coconut chutney

A creamy chutney from South India, this is particularly good served with mild curries. It will keep well in the fridge for up to 3 days.

Serves 4

8 tbsp dried, shredded coconut	1 tsp fenugreek seeds
4 tbsp yogurt	¼ fresh green chili, deseeded and finely chopped
½ tsp salt	12 curry leaves, fresh or dried
2 tsp ghee, sesame oil, or coconut oil	1 sprig fresh coriander, to garnish
2 tsp black mustard seeds	

1. Put the shredded coconut in a bowl and pour enough cold water over it to just cover. Leave to soak for about 15 minutes.

2. Blend the soaked coconut, yogurt, and salt in a blender or food processor to form a paste. Transfer to a bowl.

3. Heat the ghee or oil in a medium saucepan. Add the black mustard seeds, and as soon as they start to pop, add the fenugreek seeds, chili, and curry leaves, and fry for about 10 seconds.

4. Stir the spice mixture into the coconut-yogurt paste until thoroughly mixed. Transfer to a serving dish and garnish with a sprig of fresh coriander.

Note

- To make this chutney suitable for vegans, substitute soy or coconut yogurt for the regular yogurt.

Date and fig chutney

This hot, sweet and sour chutney keeps fresh in the fridge for up to 3 days. Dates and figs are full of fiber, essential vitamins and minerals, and antioxidants.

Serves 4

8 dates, pitted and finely chopped	3 tbsp fresh ginger, finely chopped
4 dried figs, hard stems removed and finely chopped	pinch of chili powder
2 tbsp raisins, finely chopped	4 tbsp lemon juice
	lemon slices, to garnish

1. Put the dates, figs, and raisins in a bowl and pour over enough hot water to just cover. Leave to soak for about 20 minutes. Drain if necessary.

2. Add the ginger, chili, and lemon juice to the soaked fruit and mix well. Transfer to a serving dish and garnish with lemon slices.

Mint and cilantro chutney

The astringent taste of this green chutney goes especially well with deep fried snacks and fried bread.

Serves 4

handful of fresh cilantro	12 cashew nuts, plus more to garnish
small handful of fresh mint leaves, plus sprig to garnish	pinch of chilli powder
2 tbsp lemon juice	pinch of salt
2 tsp olive oil	

1. Place all ingredients, except the mint and cashew nuts for the garnish, in a blender or food processor. Blitz, adding just enough water to form a smooth paste.

2. Transfer to a serving bowl and garnish with cashew nuts and a sprig of fresh mint.

Breads

Whole grain breads are a good source of fiber, B vitamins, and protein. If you are reluctant to eat wheat or yeast, you will be able to find alternative grains in health food shops and the recipes given here are all yeast-free.

Parathas

These simple yet delicious yeast-free breads can accompany a soup or main course, or can be eaten with a chutney as a light snack. For a gluten-free option, replace the whole wheat flour with 50 percent buckwheat flour and 50 percent rice flour.

Makes 8

9oz (250g) whole wheat flour or "chapati atta," plus extra for dusting

½ tsp salt

4 tsp ghee or oil

1. Put the flour and salt in a large bowl and mix in just enough water to form a soft, but not sticky, dough. Turn out onto a floured work surface and knead thoroughly until the dough becomes elastic. The stronger the kneading, the better the paratha. Cover the dough with a damp cloth and leave to rest for 1 hour at room temperature.

2. Divide the dough into eight equal-size balls. Lightly dust a chopping board or work surface with a little flour. Using a rolling pin, roll each dough ball out into a thin, flat round. Sprinkle with a little flour if it starts to stick to the rolling pin.

3. Brush the surface of each round of dough with a little ghee or oil and fold it in half. Brush the surface once more with ghee or oil and fold it half again, so that you have a quarter circle. Carefully roll it out into a large triangle.

4. Heat a non-stick frying pan over medium heat, add a little ghee or oil to the pan, and fry the triangles of dough for about 2-3 minutes on one side, then flip, add a little more ghee or oil to the pan, and fry the other side until cooked.

5. Serve immediately, if possible, or keep warm in the oven for up to 20 minutes.

Cillas

These savory chickpea pancakes make a delicious, protein-rich snack. If you are making a whole batch of cillas, you can keep them warm in the oven for up to 20 minutes before serving.

Makes 8

9oz (250g) chickpea flour, sifted

4 tbsp sunflower, olive, sesame, or canola oil

2 tsp salt

1 fresh green chili, deseeded and thinly sliced

4 tsp fresh ginger, finely chopped

2 tsp ground turmeric

2 tsp curry powder

4 tbsp fresh coriander, coarsely chopped

1. Place all the ingredients in a large bowl and whisk together with just enough water to form a thick batter.

2. Heat a lightly oiled, non-stick frying pan over a high heat. Reduce the heat to medium and pour one large ladle of batter into the pan. Swirl the pan so the batter spreads around evenly, and cook until it starts to solidify and turn golden brown. Flip over and cook for 1-2 minutes on the other side, drizzling a little more oil around the edges.

3. Serve hot with chutneys (see p239) and yogurt on the side.

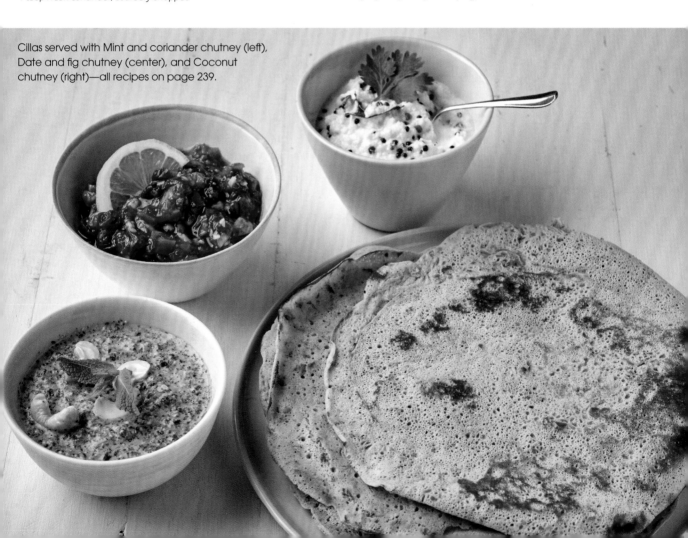

Cillas served with Mint and coriander chutney (left), Date and fig chutney (center), and Coconut chutney (right)—all recipes on page 239.

Sweet treats and desserts

Sweets should be used as occasional treats and not as staple foods. In that context, especially when served as part of a celebration or with friends and family, they should be eaten with joy, love, and an easy conscience! Using non-refined sweeteners such as cinnamon, honey, maple syrup, and coconut, rather than sugar, these dessert recipes are tasty, satisfying, and good for the soul.

Vanilla pears with a creamy filling

Here is a low-fat, vitamin-packed, refreshingly fruity dessert. You can use apples or fresh peaches, when in season, instead of the pears.

Serves 4

2 large, firm, ripe pears
2 tsp lemon juice
8 tbsp ricotta or cottage cheese
4 tbsp light raw cane sugar
2 tsp vanilla extract
½ tsp ground cinnamon, plus extra to garnish
4 whole almonds, skinned, to garnish

1. Peel the pears (leave skin on if organic), halve lengthways, and remove and discard the cores. Place the pear halves in a large saucepan and add 4 tablespoons of water. Bring to a boil, turn heat to low, and leave the pears to simmer for about 10 minutes, or until they are tender. Remove pears from the pan, sprinkle with the lemon juice, and leave to cool.

2. In a bowl, mix the cheese, sugar, vanilla extract, and cinnamon together until well blended.

3. Place each pear half in a serving dish. Top each with a quarter of the cheese mixture, and garnish with an almond and sprinkling of cinnamon. Serve.

Note

- For a vegan option, substitute the cheese with thickened soy or coconut yogurt. To thicken yogurt, line a colander or sieve with a sheet of muslin or a clean tea towel and set it over a large bowl. Put 9oz (250g) soy or coconut yogurt onto the muslin or tea towel and leave to drain for about 1 hour.

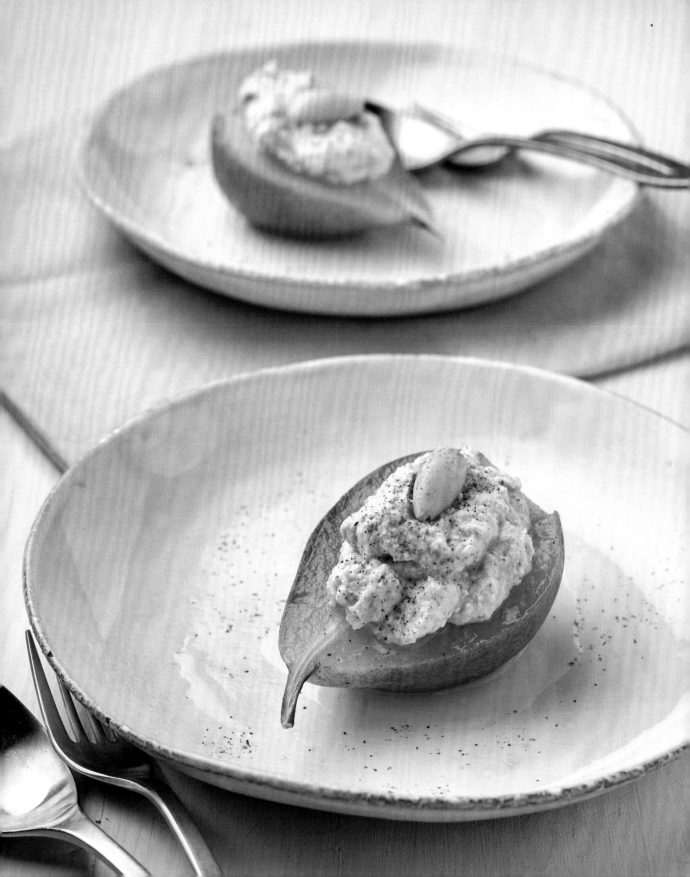

Very simple oatmeal spice cake

If you love homemade cake but are not much of a baker, try this easy vegan recipe that always turns out well. Wrapped in foil, this cake will stay fresh for up to a week.

Makes 1 cake

3oz (85g) rolled oats

4½oz (125g) wholemeal flour

5¾oz (170g) raw cane sugar

2½oz (75g) raisins

3½oz (100g) mixed chopped nuts or seeds, such as almonds, cashew nuts, hazelnuts, walnuts, sesame seeds, sunflower seeds, or shredded coconut

2 tsp baking powder

1 tsp ground cinnamon

1 tsp ground cardamom

1 tsp ground nutmeg

pinch of ground cloves

4 tbsp sunflower oil

1. Preheat the oven to 350°F (180°C/Gas 4). Lightly grease a 9in (23cm) round cake pan.

2. Place all the ingredients except the oil in a large mixing bowl and stir to mix evenly together. Create a well in the center and pour in the sunflower oil and 6fl oz (175ml) water. Mix thoroughly until well combined.

3. Pour the mixture into the greased cake pan and smooth to even out. Bake for about 45 minutes, or until a knife or metal skewer inserted in the center comes out clean. Remove from the oven and leave to cool slightly. Turn out of the pan and cool completely on a wire rack before serving.

Note

• For a gluten-free version, substitute buckwheat flour or quinoa flour for the wholemeal flour and buckwheat or millet flakes for the oats.

Chocolate muffins

These are a real treat for chocolate lovers. The addition of bananas give texture and moisture to these fabulously yummy muffins.

Makes 12

9oz (250g) wholemeal flour

2 tsp baking powder

4½oz (125g) cocoa powder

12oz (350g) raw cane sugar

2 tsp lemon juice

1 tsp vanilla powder, or vanilla essence

3 tbsp sunflower oil

3 medium, ripe bananas, mashed

For the icing

4½oz (125g) butter, or organic margarine, at room temperature

2 tbsp golden icing sugar

½ tsp vanilla extract

1. Preheat the oven to 325°F (160°C/Gas 3). Place paper liners in a 12-cup muffin pan.

2. Put the flour, baking powder, and cocoa powder in a mixing bowl and stir until evenly mixed.

3. In a separate mixing bowl, mix together the sugar, lemon juice, vanilla powder, and 10fl oz (300ml) hot water. Stir until the sugar has dissolved, then stir in the oil and the mashed bananas.

4. Fold the banana mixture into the flour mixture until the two are well combined. Divide the mixture evenly between the muffin cups and bake for 25-30 minutes, or until well risen and golden. Remove the muffins from the baking pan and cool on a wire rack.

5. Meanwhile, make the icing. Combine the butter or margarine with the sugar and vanilla extract in a mixing bowl. Once the muffins are cool, spread some icing on the top of each muffin.

Note

• For a gluten-free version, substitute a mixture of 4½oz (125g) rice flour and 4½oz (125g) buckwheat flour for the wholemeal flour.

Cardamom-ginger Highland shortbread

Serve these melt-in-the-mouth shortbread fingers with a cup of refreshing herbal tea. They make a soothing and uplifting treat at any time, but especially on a cold and wet winter afternoon.

Makes 60

12oz (350g) wholemeal flour

6oz (175g) rice flour

6oz (175g) raw cane sugar, plus extra for dusting

12oz (350g) cold butter, cut into small cubes

pinch of salt

1 tsp finely grated orange zest (preferably from an organic orange)

3 tsp ground cardamom

2 tsp ground ginger

1. Line a baking sheet with parchment paper.

2. In a large mixing bowl, combine all the ingredients. Work quickly and avoid over mixing, because this will make the shortbread tough.

3. Spread out the dough evenly on the baking sheet, so it is about ½in (1cm) thick. Place in the fridge for 1 hour.

4. Meanwhile, preheat the oven to 325°F (160°C/Gas 3). Remove the baking sheet from the fridge and with a sharp knife cut the dough on the sheet into 60 equal-size fingers. Prick the top of each finger all over with a fork.

5. Place the sheet into the oven and bake for 20–35 minutes until the shortbread is lightly golden. Remove from the oven and with a sharp knife cut the shortbread fingers again along the pre-cut lines.

6. While still hot, dust liberally with sugar. Allow to cool completely before removing from the tray and serving.

Notes

- For a gluten-free version, substitute buckwheat flour for the wholemeal flour.

- For a vegan version, use organic margarine instead of butter.

Snacks and beverages

Snacks are not recommended in yoga, as eating between meals is thought to reduce digestive capacity and place an unnecessary burden on the body. However, with the hectic schedules that many of us follow today, healthy snacks may be necessary from time to time. To avoid commercial products that are high in sugar, salt, and fat, try these easily prepared alternatives, or snack on fruit and nuts.

Open rice-paper wraps

This energizing and mouthwatering vegan snack is packed with vital vitamins and minerals, as well as being high in protein.

Makes 8

7oz (200g) baby spinach leaves

1 large, firm, ripe avocado

2 tsp lemon juice

8 rice-paper wrappers, each about 9in (23cm) in diameter

16 cherry tomatoes, halved

16 black or green olives, pitted and halved

5½oz (150g) smoked tofu, cut into 24 equal strips

4 tsp roasted sesame oil

For the dip

6 tbsp tamari

3 tsp maple syrup

pinch of chili powder

1. First prepare the dip. Combine the tamari, maple syrup, and chili powder in a small bowl. Divide equally between 4 small serving bowls and set aside.

2. To prepare the filling, divide the spinach into 8 equal portions and set aside. Halve the avocado, then remove and discard the stone and skin. Cut each avocado half into 16 slices and drizzle the lemon juice over them. Set aside.

3. Dip a rice-paper wrapper into a soup plate filled with lukewarm water for a few seconds, shake off any excess water, and put the wrapper on a cutting board or clean countertop.

4. Spread a portion of the spinach, 4 tomato halves, 4 olive halves, 3 strips of smoked tofu, and 4 slices of avocado on the wrapper. Make sure you place the filling in the middle of the wrapper, leaving about an inch clear at the edges. Drizzle with half a teaspoon of the roasted sesame oil.

5. Fold one side of the wrapper up and over the filling, then fold two other sides around the filling, one at a time, creating a tight wrap that is open at the top.

6. Repeat with the remaining 7 rice-paper wrappers and the filling ingredients to make a total of 8 wraps.

7. Serve 2 wraps per person on a small serving plate with a bowl of the dip on the side.

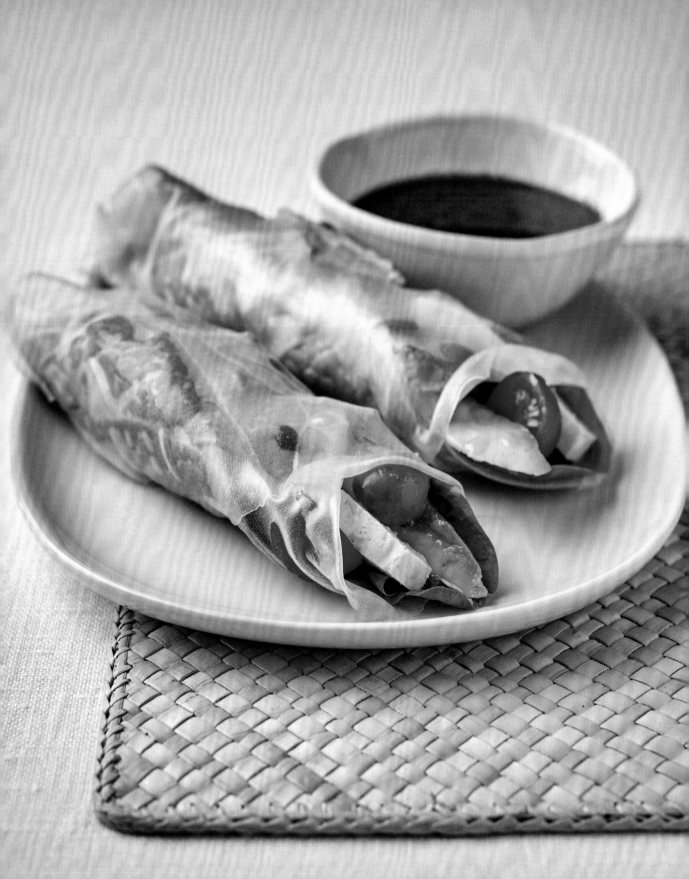

Vegetable sticks with goat's cream cheese dip

This refreshing snack will help to cool you down on a hot sunny summer afternoon. Serve with seeded whole grain Turkish flatbreads to turn it into a light lunch.

Serves 4

7oz (200g) spreadable goat's cheese

7oz (200g) yogurt, full or low fat

2 tsp lemon juice

2 tsp fresh basil, finely chopped

salt and freshly ground black pepper

4 carrots

1 cucumber

1 pepper, any color

1. Prepare the dip by the mixing the cheese, yogurt, lemon juice, basil, and salt and pepper to taste together with a fork until well combined. Set aside and keep cool.

2. Peel the carrots and cucumber and cut into chunky sticks. Halve and deseed the pepper and cut into thick slices.

3. Serve the dip with the prepared vegetables on the side.

Note

- For a vegan option, substitute the yogurt with thickened soy or coconut yogurt—see note on page 242. Use 1lb 2oz (500g) yogurt, allowing it to drain for 2 hours. You will need to season the dip with a bit more salt than the dairy version.

Guacamole

Avocados are loaded with fiber, healthy fats, and various key vitamins and minerals. Make sure you use only ripe avocados for your guacamole—the pulp inside should be tender and a rich.

Serves 4

2 ripe avocado

4 tbsp olive oil

1 pinch chili powder

4 tbsp fresh basil or fresh coriander, coarsely chopped

4 tbsp lemon juice

salt

8 black olives, pitted, to garnish

whole basil leaves or coriander sprigs, to garnish

slices of lemon, to garnish

1. Halve the avocados and remove and discard the stone and skin. Place the flesh in a bowl and mash with a fork.

2. Fold in the oil, chili powder, chopped basil or coriander, lemon juice, and salt to taste.

3. Place the mixture in a serving bowl and garnish with the olives, whole basil leaves or sprigs of coriander, and slices of lemon. Serve immediately.

Digestive lassi

It is recommended to drink a glass of this lassi every day after lunch, as it stimulates digestion. Store any extra in an airtight container in the fridge.

Serves 5

3 tsp cumin seeds
10oz (300g) full-fat yogurt
1 pint (600ml) water

salt
½ tsp ground ginger
pinch of chili powder

1. Heat a dry frying pan on medium heat, add the cumin seeds, and toast until they turn fragrant and darken slightly, but take care not to burn them. Grind the toasted seeds into powder using a pestle and mortar or an electric coffee grinder.

2. Using a whisk or a blender, mix all ingredients, including the ground cumin seeds, into a creamy drink.

Notes

- To save time, you can use store-bought ground cumin (don't toast it).
- Vegans can use soy or coconut yogurt.

Lemonade with fresh mint and orange-blossom water

Mint is a very cooling herb, so this Asian-style lemonade helps to cool down on hot days. Never drink it ice cold as it will disturb the digestive fire.

Serves 4

4 tbsp finely chopped fresh mint, plus 4 sprigs, to garnish
1¼ pints (750ml) bottled still spring water
8 tbsp lemon juice (or more, according to taste)

2 tsp orange-blossom water (or more, according to taste)
sweetener such as agave syrup, honey, or stevia, to taste
4 slices of lemon

1. Place the chopped mint in a heatproof container with a lid. Pour a little boiling water over the mint, cover, and let it brew for a few minutes. Pour through a sieve, retaining the liquid.

2. Mix the bottled spring water, the mint-flavored liquid, lemon juice, and orange-blossom water together in a large jug. Sweeten according to taste.

3. Put a sprig of fresh mint and one slice of lemon into each of 4 serving glasses, pour the lemonade over it, and serve.

Resources

International Sivananda Yoga Vedanta Centers and Ashrams
Founder: Swami Vishnudevananda

www.sivananda.org

Ashrams

HEADQUARTERS: CANADA

Sivananda Ashram Yoga Camp
673, 8th Avenue Val Morin
Quebec J0T 2R0, Canada
www.sivananda.org/camp

AUSTRIA

Sivananda Yoga Retreat House
Bichlach 40
A- 6370 Reith bei Kitzbühel
Tyrol, Austria
www.sivananda.at

BAHAMAS

Sivananda Ashram Yoga Retreat
P.O. Box N7550 Paradise Island Nassau,
Bahamas
www.sivanandabahamas.org

FRANCE

Château du Yoga Sivananda
26 Impasse du Bignon
45170 Neuville aux bois, France
www.sivanandaorleans.org

INDIA

Sivananda Yoga Vedanta
Meenakshi Ashram
Near Pavanna Vilakku Junction,
New Natham Road
Saramthangi Village
Madurai Dist. 625 503
Tamil Nadu, South India
www.sivananada.org/madurai

Sivananda Kutir
(Near Siror Bridge)
P.O. Netala, Uttar Kashi Dt,
Uttarakhand, Himalayas, 249 193,
North India
www.sivananda.org/netala

Sivananda Yoga Vedanta
Dhanwantari Ashram
P.O. Neyyar Dam
Thiruvananthapuram Dt.
Kerala, 695 572, India
www.sivananda.org/neyyardam

International Sivananda Yoga Vedanta
Tapaswini Ashram
Guthavaripalem, Kadivedu P.O.
Chilakur Mandalam,Gudur, India
www.sivananda.org.in/gudur

UNITED STATES

Sivananda Ashram Yoga Ranch
P.O. Box 195, 500 Budd Road
Woodbourne, NY 12788, USA
www.sivanandayogaranch.org

Sivananda Ashram Yoga Farm
14651 Ballantree Lane
Grass Valley, CA 95949, USA
www.sivanandayogafarm.org

VIETNAM

**Sivananda Yoga Vietnam Resort and
Training Center**
K'Lan Eco Resort
Tuyen Lam Lake;
Dalat, Vietnam
www.sivanandayogavietnam.org

Centers

ARGENTINA

**Centro Internaciónal de Yoga
Sivananda**
Sánchez de Bustamante 2372 -
(C.P. 1425)
Capital Federal - Buenos Aires -
Argentina
www.sivananda.org/buenosaires

Centro de Yoga Sivananda
Rioja 425, 8300 Neuquén
Argentina
www.facebook.com/
SivanandaNequen/

AUSTRIA

Sivananda Yoga Vedanta Zentrum
Prinz Eugen Strasse 18
A -1040 Vienna, Austria
www.sivananda.org/vienna

BRAZIL

Centro Sivananda de Yoga Vedanta
Rua Santo Antônio 374, Barrio Floresta
Porto Alegre 90220-010, Brazil
www.sivananda.org/portoalegre

**Centro International Sivananda de
Yoga e Vedanta**
Rua Girassol 1088, Vila Madalena
Sao Paulo 05433-002, Brazil
www.sivananda.org/saopaulo

CANADA

Sivananda Yoga Vedanta Center
5178 St Lawrence Blvd
Montreal
Quebec H2T 1R8, Canada
www.sivananda.org/montreal

Sivananda Yoga Vedanta Center
77 Harbord Street
Toronto
Ontario M5S 1G4, Canada
www.sivananda.org/toronto

CHINA

Sivananda Yoga Vedanta Center
Zhonghuayuan Xiuyuan 30-3-202
5 Tongzilin East Road
Wuhou District, Chengdu, Sichuan
610041, China
www.sivanandayogachina.org

FRANCE

Centre Sivananda de Yoga Vedanta
140 rue du Faubourg Saint-Martin
F-75010 Paris, France
www.sivananda.org/paris

GERMANY

Sivananda Yoga Vedanta Zentrum
Steinheilstrasse 1
D-80333 Munich, Germany
www.sivananda.org/munich

Sivananda Yoga Vedanta Zentrum
Schmiljanstrasse 24
D-12161 Berlin, Germany
www.sivananda.org/berlin

INDIA

Sivananda Yoga Vedanta Nataraja Center
A-41 Kailash Colony
New Delhi 110 048, India
www.sivananda.org/delhi

Sivananda Yoga Vedanta Dwarka Center
(near DAV school, next to Kamakshi Apts) PSP Pocket, Secor – 6
Swami Sivananda Marg,
Dwarka, New Delhi 110075, India
www.sivananda.org/dwarka

Sivananda Yoga Vedanta Center
TC37/1927 (5), Airport Road
West Fort P.O.
Thiruvananthapuram
Kerala 695 023, India
www.sivananda.org/trivandrum

Sivananda Yoga Vedanta Center
3/655 (Plot No. 131) Kaveri Nagar,
Kuppam Road, Kottivakkam
Chennai, Tamil Nadu 600 041, India
www.sivananda.org/chennai

Sivananda Yoga Vedanta Center
444, K.K. Nagar, East 9th Street
Madurai
Tamil Nadu 625 020, India
www.sivananda.org/maduraicentre

ISRAEL

Sivananda Yoga Vedanta Center
6 Lateris St
Tel Aviv 64166, Israel
www.sivananda.co.il

ITALY

Centro Yoga Vedanta Sivananda Roma
via Oreste Tommasini, 7
00162 Rome, Italy
www.sivananda-yoga-roma.it

JAPAN

Sivananda Yoga Vedanta Center
4-15-3 Koenji-kita, Suginami-ku
Tokyo 1660002, Japan
www.sivananda.jp

LITHUANIA

Šivananda Jogos Vedantos Centras Vilniuje
M.K. Čiurlionio g.66
03100 Vilnius, Lithuania
www.sivananda.org/vilnius

SPAIN

Centro de Yoga Sivananda Vedanta
Calle Eraso 4
28028 Madrid, Spain
www.sivananda.org/madrid

SWITZERLAND

Centre Sivananda de Yoga Vedanta
1 Rue des Minoteries
1205 Geneva, Switzerland
www.sivananda.org/geneva

UNITED KINGDOM

Sivananda Yoga Vedanta Center
45–51 Felsham Road
London SW15 1AZ, UK
www.sivananda.co.uk

UNITED STATES

Sivananda Yoga Vedanta Center
1246 West Bryn Mawr Avenue
Chicago, IL 60660, USA
www.sivanandachicago.org

Sivananda Yoga Vedanta Center
243 West 24th Street
New York, NY 10011, USA
www.sivanandanyc.org

Sivananda Yoga Vedanta Center
1185 Vincente Street
San Francisco, CA 94122, USA
www.sivanandasf.org

Sivananda Yoga Vedanta Center
13325 Beach Avenue
Marina del Rey, CA 90292, USA
www.sivanandala.org

URUGUAY

Asociación de Yoga Sivananda
Acevedo Díaz 1523
11200 Montevideo, Uruguay
www.sivananda.org/montevideo

VIETNAM

Sivananda Yoga Vedanta Center
25 Tran Quy Khoach Street, District 1
Ho Chi Minh City, Vietnam
www.sivanandayogavietnam.org

Index

Acknowledgments

About the authors

The International Sivananda Yoga Vedanta Centers were established in 1957 by Swami Vishnudevananda (1927–1993). This nonprofit organization with locations around the world is dedicated to the teaching of classical yoga and vedanta philosophy as a way to promote physical, mental, and spiritual health.

As part of a global network of ashrams and centers, yoga teachers guide their students in developing an integral practice of yoga and meditation. More than 46,000 yoga teachers have graduated from the international Sivananda teachers' training courses since 1969.

The authors of this book are Swami Durgananda, Swami Sivadasananda, and Swami Kailasananda. They were personally trained by Swami Vishnudevananda as Yoga Acharyas (senior teachers) and are members of the Executive Board of the International Sivananda Yoga Organization. www.sivananda.org

Author's acknowledgments

The Sivananda Yoga Vedanta Center would like to thank Prema, Satyadev, and Liese for their skill and enthusiasm in demonstrating the yoga techniques; Hilary Mandleberg for the skilful editing work; Swami Bhagavatananda for the delicious and healthy recipes; and the very dedicated and enthusiastic team at DK.

To find out more about the Sivananda Yoga Vedanta Centers go to: www.sivananda.org or contact Swami Sivadasananda, e-mail: sws@sivananda.net

Publisher's acknowledgments

Dorling Kindersley would like to thank John Freeman for all the model photography; models Prema (Karina Andrea Arenas Bonansea), Satyadev (Steeve Petteau), and Liese Grillmayer; Rachel Jones for hair and makeup; Kevin Boak of Kevin Boak Studio; the Sivananda Yoga Vedanta center, London, for the loan of props and mats; William Reavell for food photography: Jane Lawrie for food styling; Rob Merrett for food prop styling; designers Nicky Collings, Mandy Earey, Anne Fisher, Ruth Hope, Helen McTeer; Danaya Bunnag for design assistance; Susannah Marriott for additional editorial help; Annelise Evans for proofreading; Hilary Bird for the original 2010 index; and Peter Bull Arts Studio for the anatomical artworks.

First edition

Project Editor Hilary Mandleberg; **Senior Editor** Jennifer Latham; **Senior Art Editor** Susan Downing; **Designers** Danaya Bunnag, Caroline de Souza, Mandy Earey, Anne Fisher, Helen McTeer; **Managing Editor** Dawn Henderson; **Managing Art Editor** Christine Keilty; **Art Director** Peter Luff; **Publisher** Mary-Clare Jerram; **DTP Designer** Sonia Charbonnier; **Senior; Production Controller** Alice Holloway; **Senior Production Editor** Ben Marcus; **Ilustrations** Peter Bull Arts Studio

Picture credits

p9 Sivananda Yoga Vendata Center
p200 (second left) Dorling Kindersley (c) Angus Beare
All other images © Dorling Kindersley
For further information see www.dkimages.com